Psychology for Health Fitness Professionals

James Gavin
Nettie Gavin

Human Kinetics

Library of Congress Cataloging-in-Publication Data

Gavin, James, 1942-
  Psychology for health fitness professionals / James Gavin and
Nettie Gavin.
    p. cm.
  Includes index.
  ISBN 0-87322-775-1 (softcover)
  1. Personal trainers--Psychology.   2. Interpersonal relations.
I. Gavin, Nettie, 1942-   . II. Title.
GV428.7.G38   1995
613.7'11'019--dc20   94-23549
                                                               CIP

ISBN: 0-87322-775-1

Acquisitions Editor: Richard D. Frey, PhD; **Developmental Editors:** Lori Garrett, Ann Brodsky, Glennda Kouts; **Assistant Editors:** Jacqueline Blakley, Anna Curry, Julie Ohnemus, and Myla Smith; **Copyeditor:** Barbara Bergstrom; **Proofreader:** John Wentworth; **Indexer:** indi-indexers; **Production Manager:** Kris Ding; **Typesetting and Text Layout:** Yvonne Winsor; **Text Designer:** Stuart Cartwright; **Cover Designer:** Jack Davis; **Printer:** United Graphics

Printed in the United States of America   10 9 8 7 6 5 4 3 2

Human Kinetics
Web site: http://www.humankinetics.com/

United States: Human Kinetics, P.O. Box 5076, Champaign, IL 61825-5076
1-800-747-4457
e-mail: humank@hkusa.com

Canada: Human Kinetics, Box 24040, Windsor, ON N8Y 4Y9
1-800-465-7301 (in Canada only)
e-mail: humank@hkcanada.com

Europe: Human Kinetics, P.O. Box IW14, Leeds LS16 6TR, United Kingdom
(44) 1132 781708
e-mail: humank@hkeurope.com

Australia: Human Kinetics, 57A Price Avenue, Lower Mitcham, South Australia 5062
(088) 277 1555
e-mail: humank@hkaustralia.com

New Zealand: Human Kinetics, P.O. Box 105-231, Auckland 1
(09) 523 3462
e-mail: humank@hknewz.com

to true love . . .
(. . . just keep on clickin')

CONTENTS

"With everything that we do in this life, the most important ingredient is the spirit with which it is done. Spirit is formed from the transformation of the energy of our experiences. Consciously directing our spirit creates enthusiasm and results in a complete participation in the present. . . . When we become solely focused on technique or results, our activities become mechanical and lifeless. When we utilize techniques and enjoy the process of their use as a vehicle for the expression of spirit, then what we are doing, regardless of what it is called, gives us a feeling of being alive, happy, and light. . . . We always have the opportunity to develop and express our spirit for life."

—Saul Goodman

PREFACE

Hello! We'd like to get to know you and have you know us. That will be a bit difficult, but you at least can get to know us here on this page, and the picture of us on page 121 gives you some faces to associate with the words.

Maybe you're sitting in a comfortable chair somewhere beginning to read our book. Or maybe you're standing in a bookstore, trying to figure out whether to buy it. Either way, let us begin with a few questions:

First, what do you do? That's a pretty broad question to start with, so we'll break it down: Are you involved in the field of health and wellness? Or do you work with fitness and sports? If you answered yes to either of these, we want you to know that we have written this book especially for you. How much time do you spend interacting with people? Maybe you work with clients or students or athletes for whom you provide a service like training, health promotion, or "hands-on" therapy. The more time you spend with people, the more you will relish the information we provide.

Second, would you like to learn some practical skills for successful professional relationships? You might want to know how practical we mean. Would you like to learn how to *capture the spirit of effective relationships*? We'll teach you how to support people in getting exactly what they need to do their very best while at the same time keeping yourself in top psychological shape. We hope you're still with us and that you've answered a definite yes to these questions.

Finally, would you like to learn how to maximize the personal resources and energies you spend on others while still having plenty for yourself?

Though it may seem a tall order to fill, we are confident we can help you do precisely that. There is work involved, yet the payoffs are worth it. The process involves a journey of insight, evaluation, and skill building. We'll show you how to care for yourself as you care for others, and how to make that your secret to success. You can expect to gain confidence in previously frustrating or difficult situations. Listening, advising, facing conflict, and providing inspiration will become your strengths.

Now that you have answered some of our questions, we'd like to tell you why we believe so strongly in what we are offering you. We bring to this book a combined wisdom accumulated over 100 years of living (that's for the two of us, of course). As further proof of our conviction about this book, we wrote it—each sentence and paragraph—together and we practiced all along the way what we advocate for you, the reader. Authorship gave us many opportunities to readjust our skills not only as writers, but also as people in relationship and as health and fitness professionals. At the end of this process, we are doing much better than when we started. Through this book we, too, have learned how to be the very best of ourselves and how we can share that with others. Corny though it may sound, we discovered we were more than our knowledge, more than our roles, more than our goals, and more than our relationship. We discovered in ourselves a place from which we were capable of being inspirational, and we are writing you from that place.

You can carry this book in one word that will bring magic to your work. The word will reveal your path to success, will give you the winning edge in a game with no losers, will enhance all dimensions of your life. The word is **SPIRIT**—the one you have and the one you want to share with others.

Read on. In this book you'll find vital answers that caring, committed people have about working with others: how to get to know them and understand what they need, how to help them meet their needs without taking responsibility for them, and how to keep yourself whole in the process.

We know that health and fitness is about the whole person, not just the body and not just the mind. And we know the whole person incorporates a special quality known mostly in moments of extraordinary human endeavor: persistence toward seemingly unreachable goals, transformations in life direction, and simple acts of profound courage.

We believe this special quality is **SPIRIT**—and it can be present in all moments of life, not just extraordinary ones. We would like to show you how to bring **SPIRIT** more fully into your work, into your relationships, and into your connection with yourself.

This book is all about capturing the **SPIRIT** in relationships. Although this word may have a unique meaning for you, we trust our meanings will blend. At its core, **SPIRIT** is about the best of you. Merging with mind and body, it allows for the actualization of your full potential.

SPIRIT unfolds in the following six chapters. Each letter of the word **SPIRIT** represents something unique and important for you and your work with others:

S stands for SUPPORT.

P represents PURPOSE.

I means INTEGRITY.

R is about RESOLUTION.

I reveals INSPIRATION.

T concerns TIMING.

Each element of **SPIRIT** is presented in two forms: theory and practice. This format provides you with the reasons for action and essential skills for doing it.

- **Support:** Chapter 1 is about being supportive to another and to yourself at the same time. Much of your work is about supporting others in their pursuit of health, wellness, and physical activity from a perspective that honors the whole person.

- **Purpose:** In health, wellness, and physical activity, we talk about short- and long-term goals and also about purpose: What do we want for our lives or in this moment? This is the core of Chapter 2. Everyone has a purpose, even though he or she may not be clear about it or know how to pursue it. Your work involves helping people discover what they want and enabling them to pursue their goals. The more ways you have of getting to that essential discussion of purpose and goals, the easier your work will be, and the more success you'll achieve.

- **Integrity:** Boundaries, such as lanes in the pool, lines on the field, rules for the game, are important in athletic pursuits. Different types of boundaries are also critical in human affairs. You need to know where you stop and someone else begins, who's responsible for what, and what rules to play by. Integrity is about defining your boundaries and limits and about respecting the other person's needs and limits. Integrity determines your personal code of conduct. This is the stuff of Chapter 3.

- **Resolution:** Conflicts are inevitable in life, and learning how to effectively resolve them will be an essential key to your success. In Chapter 4 we'll help you understand conflict, appreciate the dynamics of power, and learn strategies for achieving mutually satisfying solutions.

- **Inspiration:** You probably know what it's like to feel inspired. Is it possible to give that to others? In Chapter 5 we'll offer you guidelines for affirming yourself as you help others tune into their own inspirational channels. You will learn how to be there for others without having to take responsibility for them. We'll show you how treating yourself with respect, understanding, caring, and fairness can generate all the inspirational energy you need for your work with others.

- **Timing:** It's all about time—performance, healing, life in general. There are times to speak and times to listen; times to act and times to wait; times to rush and times to relax. Knowing how to determine when is what timing is all about, and in Chapter 6 we'll present some straightforward principles about when and when not to . . .

Are you ready? Then may we suggest that you turn the page.

ACKNOWLEDGMENTS

The SPIRIT of this book came from many sources in our present lives and throughout our histories. To fully acknowledge the people and experiences that have inspired, supported, and loved us along the way would take up far more space than our publisher would allow. We wish to thank some special wizards who in so many different ways have shown us who we really are and celebrated with us: Nettie's parents, Helen and Louis Spector; Jim's birth parents, Mary and Paddy Gavin; and his "adopted" parents, Dick and Margaret McDonald; our siblings and their wives, Tom and Joanna Spector, Pat and Patty Gavin, and Maureen "A." Gavin; our magical children, David Glickman, Geoffrey Glickman, Jessica Gavin, Jacob Gavin, and Susannah Gavin; and Charlie the cat. We love you as much as we say we do, and we have been deeply touched by your caring and encouragement.

True love doesn't grow on trees, yet writing this book helped water, fertilize, and nurture ours. According to Nettie, Jim (aka "Gav") encouraged the evolution and expression of her ideas, lived through lively debates around power, and understood her determination to sneak as much love as possible into the book. His gifts of humor and playfulness added to the heart of this book. According to Gav, Nettie (aka "Natasha") enabled him to walk his talk—and write from the heart. Her loving touch and inner knowing can be felt as much as seen throughout the pages.

Chapter 1

SUPPORT:
BEING PRESENT IN POSITIVE WAYS

"One need not love everyone—one need only act lovingly toward others."

—Martin Buber

The second class of the Health for Life program at the local YMCA was off to a great start. The instructor, a cherubic-looking man in his mid-40s, had just asked participants for progress reports about the lifestyle commitments they had made in the first session.

Diane was describing how her family reacted to her "lifestyle improvements." She was on a roll, like a stand-up comic on amateur night. "Well, my father said it was about time. Then he added, 'You should have done this a long time ago when I told you to.' My mother seemed hurt, especially when I told her I wanted to try out some new recipes. My older sister made it all sound so simple. She said, 'If you just watch what you eat like I do and take fitness classes with me, you'll be perfectly healthy.' Then, there was Ernie, my little brother. I think I got the most support from him. He said, 'Go for it, Sis. Live long and prosper.'

"You have to understand," Diane added with a twinkle. "Ernie's a Trekkie."

Sam was next to jump into the feedback session with his version of "Change Meets Godzilla." Sam's commitment to healthy eating met its first challenge at work the day after the first session. It was break time, and he had just gotten his order from the coffee wagon. Sean saw him munching on an apple and asked, "Hey, Sam, what's wrong? No donuts this morning?" When Sam tried to explain, Sean cut him off with a loud announcement: "Hey, guys, Sam here has gone bananas; he's gonna be a health food nut." Dennis tried to offer some support. "Hey, give Sam a break. The way he eats, Sam's his own worst enemy." Sally watched Sam wince at this comment and came to his defense. "We all have crummy eating habits in this office. Sam's not nearly as bad as the rest of you."

Fortunately, Sam reported, the situation improved the next day. He found a small brown bag on his desk with one ripe, red apple and a note: "Way to go, Sam—Billy."

Pete, resembling a Zen monk sitting in his chair, was next with his story. "Well, as you all know, I decided last week I was going to try 20 minutes of meditation every morning before work. I took the pamphlet from class and showed it to my wife. She couldn't understand why I needed to meditate. She said I looked like I was in a coma most mornings anyway. My father told me if I thought I had stress, I should have been with him in Korea. I think the only real support I got was from my dog, Daisy. When I got myself all set to meditate each morning, she came and sat quietly beside me—even her breathing helped me get into it."

This story is about support—what some people understand support to be and, on the receiving end, what real support feels like. Perhaps you can identify with some of the characters in this story. You may have experienced trying to change something in your life and having friends and family rush to offer support—what they thought was support. Their intentions were probably good, yet they may have gotten sidetracked in the delivery.

CORE CONDITIONS FOR SUPPORT

Being supportive is more difficult than might seem apparent. We discuss its components in this section so you can fully appreciate them. There are three core conditions for supporting someone:

- Being fully receptive to the person
- Acknowledging the person's words and feelings without judgment
- Offering assistance appropriate to your role, your resources, and the situation (RRS)

We will illustrate these core conditions by describing supportive interactions in settings you're likely to recognize. We will also identify the benefits of being supportive.

The first thing to know about support is that it isn't all or nothing. You can offer people degrees of support. Sometimes your presence alone can comfort another person in a strange or frightening situation.

The more open you are to receiving another person, the more you acknowledge—without judgment—his or her communications. The more you provide appropriate kinds and levels of assistance, the more that person will experience your support.

CONDITION 1: *Being Fully Receptive*

Think about how you feel when you talk to someone who is half listening. Hurt? Unimportant? Angry?

Full support demands your full attention. The listener must put personal issues temporarily aside. To be fully receptive, you'll want to clear your mind as best you can and to listen without filtering, without interpreting, and without holding expectations.

Being fully receptive means doing only one thing in the moment: committing yourself to the interaction (see Figure 1.1). It means putting away papers you're working on so they won't distract you, shutting off the telephone so you aren't interrupted, and quieting yourself down so the other person can feel your attention.

You might think we're asking the impossible. When 10 people are lined up to talk to you, how can you give anyone your undivided attention? A partial answer lies in the distinction between quality and quantity. Five minutes of your focused presence may be worth 50 minutes of diluted attention.

Body language helps communicate your support. Your presence becomes known to the other person the more you allow your eyes to meet, the more receptive you allow your body to be, and the more you allow yourself to breathe. Yes, breathe. Whenever you tense up, you typically interrupt your normal rhythm of breathing.

Figure 1.1

What "Being Fully Receptive" Looks Like

Meeting the other's eyes	**not**	Staring or shifting your eyes
Facing the person	**not**	Turning sideways or away
Focusing your attention	**not**	Allowing distractions
Quieting your body rhythms	**not**	Yielding to impatience
Opening your body posture	**not**	Closing yourself off (arms folded across chest, frown on your face, head tilted in doubt)

We're not suggesting you rivet yourself in place and stare at someone with a fixed gaze. Being present to another comes from being present in yourself: taking a deep breath and letting go of extraneous thoughts as you exhale; relaxing your muscles in the moment so your body is free to receive impressions, rather than prepared to evaluate them; slowing down enough to take in what's happening.

CONDITION 2: *Acknowledging Words and Feelings*

You may think that when someone tells you about a problem, you have to do something to fix it or perhaps that you have to agree with her perspective on it. Acknowledging a person's words and feelings is quite straightforward. It means hearing what someone says to you and being aware of her feelings without taking personal responsibility for them and without judging the supposed rightness or wrongness of her communication.

At some point in your conversation, you may need to make a judgment about the situation or to take some responsibility for it. Even so, enhancing your communication skills starts with unfiltered awareness of the other person's experience. If you put yourself into an evaluative mode or a responsibility-taking position at the outset, you may misinterpret the other person's needs or intentions.

The following scenario illustrates some common errors identifiable in the responses we make to another person's communication.

A Potential Client on Her First Visit to a Health and Fitness Center

Imagine you are a staff trainer at a health and fitness center. You observe an overweight woman huffing and puffing as she climbs the stairs toward your reception area. After about 5 minutes of introductions and explanations, Carol, the potential client, offers her reasons for coming:

> **Carol:**
>
> "My friends keep telling me I should join a health club. They say I'm overweight and out of shape. . . . I don't think I'm that overweight, do you? . . . And I'm sure I can run faster than most of them. [Pauses with a deep sigh] It really galls me to hear them passing judgment on me! But anyway, here I am. . . . So what do you think you can do for me?"

A staff trainer might make any of the following six common errors when attempting to acknowledge Carol's words and feelings.

- **Denying response:** "Carol, I don't think you're overweight. . . . You seem to be in pretty good shape to me. Even so, getting regular exercise is important to everyone."

  When we see that another person is upset, we may want to do whatever we think is necessary to relieve that person's discomfort—including denying what may be the truth. Carol's puffing up the stairs suggests she may be out of shape, and she appears overweight. Denying the severity of someone's problems may help temporarily, but in the long run, it goes against both your interests.

- **Agreeing response:** "Carol, I agree. If you weren't carrying those extra pounds, you might not be huffing and puffing coming up those stairs. . . . Your friends have a point, and they're probably just looking out for your best interests."

  This comment may sound honest, but it's more than that. It's agreeing with certain attitudes and perceptions based on minimal information. We've said that Carol appears out of shape and overweight, but the response has two potential problems. First, Carol may have run a few blocks before she reached your club, so she might not be as out of shape as she first seems. Second, Carol may not be entirely ready to face herself. She criticizes her friends and asks you to deny their perceptions ("I don't think I'm that overweight, do you?"). Agreeing with her friends' perceptions immediately puts you on their side against her. We believe people need to "own" their problems. Confirming what may seem obvious doesn't always help. People need to accept their problems as their own, not as the biased perceptions of others.

- **Minimizing response:** "Carol, don't worry—a lot of people could shed a few extra pounds. Recent studies show almost 65% of adults are at least 5 pounds overweight. . . . And we can all work on getting more fit, can't we now?"

This response may seem supportive because it minimizes Carol's problems. It generalizes her weight concerns to the majority of the population. In effect, you tell Carol she's not alone—her excess weight is not so bad. This response has two problematic aspects: It doesn't address her feelings (you tell her not to worry), and it voices implicit agreement with all the people she believes are attacking her. You side with her critics. She may smile and say something like "I guess you're right," while inside she may begin to feel more upset.

- **Responsibility-taking response:** "Carol, don't feel bad. If you join this club, we'll get you into a regular exercise program, and we'll make sure you lose weight and shape up in no time."

This response contains flaws similar to the previous one. It ignores Carol's feelings and implicitly agrees with her critics. It goes one step further, however, by indicating that you are taking responsibility for solving her problem. You're going to "fix" her—and if she doesn't lose weight and shape up, it's going to be your fault.

- **Blaming response:** "Well, Carol, it really doesn't matter what your friends say. . . . What matters is that you've let yourself go, and it's time to do something about it."

It may be hard to imagine saying something with such an intense quality of blaming Carol. "You have no one to blame but yourself!" is your core message. Even though you might be right, Carol would feel so criticized by this response that she might be shamed into joining your club—and then never show up again.

- **Avoiding response:** "Carol, let me tell you more about our club, and maybe that'll give you a better idea of what you can accomplish here."

This response ignores Carol's remarks—she becomes invisible. Your message may come across as "What you're telling me isn't important!" You don't always have to acknowledge the importance of someone's comment with words. You can pause reflectively to signal that you've heard what she said. This comment, however, shows no acknowledgment of Carol's feelings or her request for reassurance.

So far, we have identified what support isn't. We suggested six possible responses that we believe are unsupportive. Through these examples we were saying that support is not

- disagreeing or denying ("You don't have a problem."),
- agreeing ("You sure are uncoordinated!"),
- minimizing the problem ("That's not so bad."),
- taking responsibility ("I can fix that for you!"),
- blaming ("Well, it's your own fault."), or
- avoiding ("Let me tell you a funny story.").

While it may be clear how avoiding and blaming would be perceived as unsupportive, it is perhaps more difficult to understand why minimizing the problem or assuring the person that you will take care of her is also considered unsupportive. Here's our reasoning. If someone is discussing a problem and you are figuring out whether you agree or how you should help, your mind will be working hard to absorb, interpret, and evaluate what you are hearing. As a result, you may not be able to listen nonjudgmentally. You may be busy finding your place in the other person's problem!

Some people may want you to fix their problems or to agree with them, but how helpful to them is that type of assistance in the long run? Imagine that each time a person struggles to lift a barbell, you rush over and lift it for him. How will this help him develop his own strength? Being supportive means trusting that the other person has the resources to solve his problem. Your support helps him access these resources.

If your style is to feel responsible for others' problems, you may tend to blame the other person for the difficulty she is experiencing, to minimize the severity of the situation, or to avoid the matter altogether. This is your understandable defense against taking on another load.

If you can listen without taking on the role of rescuer and if you can separate yourself from the very real feelings another person expresses—even when they are directed at you—you will be better able to acknowledge the person's experience without judging it. This in itself will be helpful.

So, what would a supportive (acknowledging) response for Carol sound like? Here are a few possibilities.

> "Carol, I hear you. It probably doesn't feel too good when friends say these things. I'd like to know how you see the situation and what ideas you might have about how I can work with you to reach your goals."

> "Carol, it seems those comments upset you. [Pause] Let me make it clear that I'm here to help you achieve your goals, not someone else's . . . so why don't we start with what you think and what you want?"

> "Carol, what I can do for you depends very much on what you want. You've told me what your friends think, and those comments seem to upset you. Can you tell me what you think and what you want?"

Two Practice Scenes for Condition 2: Acknowledging Without Judgment

To help you distinguish real support from mistaken interpretations of support, we would like you to examine the following scenes involving health/fitness professionals. Consider each of the responses to understand the differences between a supportive (acknowledging) response and less helpful replies.

Situation A: Physiotherapy Patient. Annette takes physiotherapy three times a week to regain strength and flexibility in an injured leg. She comes regularly but doesn't work very hard. She reproaches you, the therapist, during a session:

Annette:

> "I'm really bummed about these sessions. I've been coming here for 2 months, and I still can't bend this knee very much. I thought someone told me I could expect results in 6 weeks!"

Unsupportive Responses

- **Blaming response:** "Annette, I didn't tell you that! Maybe you heard it wrong—I can't imagine anyone here saying that. . . . Have you thought about working harder during your sessions?''

- **Denying response:** ''Listen, Annette, there's really nothing to be upset about. Most people with your problem would be thrilled to have made the progress you have.''

- **Avoiding response:** ''Hey Annette, don't worry. Besides I wanted to show you a new machine we got today. You'll like it. . . . It's fun.''

- **Taking responsibility:** ''Annette, I think I know what we're doing wrong. I'm going to spend some extra time with you in the next few sessions to make sure we're helping you the way we should.''

- **Agreeing response:** ''Yeah, Annette, I guess we've let you down. . . . I don't see much improvement either.''

- **Minimizing response:** ''Annette, you're making a mountain out of a molehill. Sure, you may not have progressed as much as you wanted to, but what do you expect for your condition?''

Supportive Responses

- ''Annette, you sound really bummed. . . . I'd like to hear more about this.''

- ''Annette, I hear you . . . and I can see how upset you are. Tell me more.''

- ''Annette, that must feel really upsetting! After 2 months, you feel you've made no progress— even though someone told you that you could see results in 6 weeks.''

- ''Annette, I hear you . . . and if I felt that way, I'd be pretty darned frustrated, too.''

You may wonder what is so magical about supportive responses that makes them better than the others. Remember that Annette comes to physiotherapy regularly but doesn't work very hard. You may think, ''It's her own fault that she hasn't gotten better." Maybe so, but your being right won't help her work harder. By responding supportively, you acknowledge Annette's feelings. You also let her know that you have heard her complaint. Most important, you create an atmosphere of trust where Annette can feel your openness, your lack of criticism, and your nondefensive attitude. You haven't taken the bait to rescue or retaliate. You have laid the groundwork for helping Annette understand what she has to do to achieve the results she desires. Ultimately, you enable her to assume responsibility for her own progress even though, in the moment, she appears to be blaming you.

Situation B: Personal Training Client.   The next scenario involves a potential client in his initial interview with a personal trainer.

Harry:

"Why am I here? Well, I guess I should get in better shape. Yeah. . . . Some of the guys in my softball league have been razzing me about slowing down."

Unsupportive Responses

- **Blaming response:** "Yeah, I bet. What do you expect carrying all that extra weight around—and those cigarettes don't help either."

- **Taking responsibility:** "Well Harry, don't worry, you've come to the right place. I'll have you shaped up in no time. Six months with me and you'll give Carl Lewis a run for his money."

- **Minimizing response:** "Harry, that's no big deal. Most people come to me with worse problems, and anyhow everyone slows down as they get older."

- **Agreeing response:** "Well, Harry, you're right. You look overweight and are probably way out of shape."

- **Denying response:** "Heck, they don't know what they're talking about. You look in great shape to me."

- **Avoiding response:** "Harry, tell me about what you do for a living."

Supportive Responses

- "Well Harry, sounds like you think you should get in better shape because the guys have been giving you a hard time."

- "Yeah, Harry, I bet that hurt to hear that. The guys on my basketball team used to call me Lead Legs."

- "Wow, that's rough, Harry, even if you agree with them."

Harry may not be showing how upset he is about such concerns as aging, peer group pressure, a declining sense of vitality, and maybe even his manliness. It would be easy to consider his remark superficial, and to brush by it to get down to business. By acknowledging Harry's feelings and letting him know you hear him, you allow him an opportunity to expand on his motives for exercising. He may choose to leave things at this level or even to minimize his feelings, but he will experience your support and validation.

The Benefits of Being Supportive

What do you gain as a health/fitness professional by acknowledging a person's feelings and concerns? Supportive responses help you create a positive climate for conversation and problem-solving. You build the other person's self-esteem by giving him your undivided and unbiased attention. By enhancing the other person's sense of self, you may enable him to deal more honestly with himself, rather than hiding behind such emotions as shame, fear, or anger. The more you accept another through supportive responses, the more that person may be able to accept himself.

Most important, people welcome supportive feedback, because it makes them feel good! You will feel good, too, when you notice your positive effect on others.

Key Point: *Acknowledging another's thoughts and feelings does not mean you agree with them.*

CONDITION 3: *Offering Appropriate Assistance*

Some interactions require only your acknowledgment. If someone says, "I've had a bad day," you don't need to promise her that you're going to turn everything around. Rather, you might respond compassionately with a statement like "Sorry to hear that."

A health/fitness professional enters into many interactions that require more than listening. When to move from acknowledgment of feelings to offers of assistance can best be decided within the framework of your role. What is your job in enabling the person to achieve his or her health or fitness goals?

Interactions typically occur in a context that defines who is responsible for what. For answering the question, "What kind of support will I offer this person?" we offer you three guidelines. They are your **R**ole, your **R**esources, and the **S**ituation. Throughout this book we shall refer to these terms as the RRS formula to guide you in deciding what's appropriate in your work with others.

Let's explore the meaning of these terms.

- **Your role:** What are you responsible for in this situation? What are the parameters of your job? What were you hired for? What was your agreement with the person who hired you?

- **Your resources:** What are you trained to do? What are your personal needs and limitations? What support systems and facilities are available to you?

- **The situation:** Is this a routine, predictable situation governed by normal expectations for your role? Or does something unique about the situation require you to behave beyond normal resource or role boundaries? For example, is it an emergency or crisis?

Role Responsibility in an Unusual Situation

You are a bodyworker midway through a shiatsu session when your client begins crying and talking about an abusive relationship. What are you trained and qualified to do in this situation? Unless you are a certified psychotherapist, your response needs to be limited to one of empathy and compassion.

Even though the situation may pull you to do more than provide support and empathy, your role demands that you remain within its boundaries and not take on the activities of a counselor or therapist. At an appropriate time in the session, your resources come into play. If you know the names of qualified professionals, you can comfortably refer your client to them.

Two Practice Scenes for Condition 3: Offering Appropriate Assistance

If the supportive responses that we recommended in the cases of Annette and Harry left you unsatisfied, it's understandable. Neither dialog would likely have ended with your initial response. Your replies acknowledged Annette and Harry without judgment. You were receptive, and you heard what each person said to you. Your next response develops out of the RRS formula—your **R**ole, your **R**esources, and the **S**ituation.

Situation A: Physiotherapy Patient. Let's pick up the interaction with Annette after you have made a supportive (acknowledging) response to her. Remember that Annette's attendance at physiotherapy is good, but she doesn't work hard in her sessions.

> *Annette:* "I'm really bummed about these sessions. I've been coming for 2 months, and I still can't bend this knee very much. I thought someone told me I could see results in 6 weeks!"
>
> *Physiotherapist:* "Annette, you sound really bummed. . . . I'd like to hear more about this."
>
> *Annette:* "Well, I'm feeling discouraged. I expected big improvements. . . . Maybe I should find another physiotherapy clinic."

Before responding to Annette's comment, think about your role, your resources, and the demands of the situation. Even though Annette is threatening to quit physiotherapy, the situation isn't an emergency or crisis. This means no extraordinary measures are necessary. You can guide your response by the normal limitations of your role and your resources.

Option 1: Assume you are a physiotherapist who has just begun working with Annette because Annette changed her schedule and her previous therapist couldn't adjust her hours.

> *New Physiotherapist:* "Annette, that's one option, yet I have another suggestion. Let's review what your goals were, what you have done so far, and let's see what we can plan together to help you achieve them now."

Option 2: Now imagine you are the physiotherapist who has been working directly with Annette over the past 2 months

> *Original Physiotherapist:* "Annette, I remember telling you that you could see results in 6 weeks, and I still stand behind that statement. Before you quit working with me, I'd like an opportunity to tell you what I think is standing in the way of your reaching your goal."
>
> *Annette:* "All right, go ahead."

Original Physiotherapist: "I truly empathize with your frustration. I also believe that for whatever reason you are not exerting the amount of effort needed to see results. So no matter what I do, unless your effort level in these sessions increases, you'll continue to be frustrated."

Annette: "So, you're telling me it's all my fault."

Original Physiotherapist: "I wouldn't label it fault, Annette. I'm just trying to be clear about what responsibilities each of us has in this situation."

These responses are framed within the boundaries of the physiotherapist's role and resources. The therapist acknowledges Annette's feelings and her proposed alternative (going to another clinic) without blame but also suggests other possibilities that fall within the therapist's role responsibilities.

Situation B: Personal Training Client.   The next scenario builds upon the one involving Harry, a potential client in an initial interview with a personal trainer.

Harry: "Why am I here? Well, I guess I should get in better shape. Yeah. . . . Some of the guys in my softball league have been razzing me about slowing down."

Trainer: "Well Harry, sounds like you think you should get in better shape because the guys have been giving you a hard time."

Harry: "Yeah, but it's okay . . . they're right . . . I should get in better shape. . . . And I know my smoking doesn't help. . . . I really ought to stop. . . . Boy, you really have your work cut out for you."

Your acknowledgment of Harry pays off. He owns his problem and adds the issue of his smoking. But then he puts the responsibility of fixing him back on you. This is the perfect opportunity to spell out your respective roles and responsibilities in a supportive response.

Trainer: "Harry, it's good to know you're personally motivated to get into better shape . . . and I'm glad you know that smoking is a problem. [Pause] Let's talk about what each of us can do in this situation."

Harry: "Okay, I'm listening."

Trainer: "I suggest working with you two or three times a week for hourly sessions. I'll design a program with you that will help you reach realistic goals. . . . Your side of the agreement is to come prepared to work at these sessions and to continue working at some aerobic activity on the days when we don't meet. . . . Harry, the smoking problem isn't something I feel best qualified to deal with.

I would strongly suggest you look into a program to help you quit. . . . Your progress with me will be affected by your smoking . . . and what you do about your smoking is up to you.''

In this response, the trainer makes clear his responsibilities and role limitations. He also identifies Harry's responsibilities and provides support—with clear boundaries.

Support or Rescue

We would like to distinguish between the words support and rescue. Support can be unconditional and limitless. When offering support you can listen to the person with full acceptance, allowing him or her all the room necessary to feel and to tell you his or her story. Rescuing a person is another matter entirely. You have professional and personal limitations on your ability to rescue, and there are some good reasons why this form of help isn't always helpful.

Doing too much for another person can create dependency instead of fostering independence. Some people may feel better if you make decisions for them or take their problems away, but in the long run such rescue activities can backfire. When your advice or assistance works, you will be a hero; when your suggestions or help fails, you will shoulder the burden.

Key Point: *Support others within the boundaries of your responsibilities in the relationship, your resources at the time, and the demands of the situation.*

SKILL DEVELOPMENT FOR SUPPORT: MIRRORING COMMUNICATIONS

Jerry, a participant in a weight management clinic, tells his nutritionist, ''I'm really having a hard time sticking to the eating plan we set up. . . . I'm sorry . . . I know I should try harder, but I seem to be my own worst enemy. I don't know what's wrong with me. I'll get back on track, I guess.''

What is Jerry really saying? Emotionally, he sounds discouraged, self-rejecting, and unfocused. Jerry has hit the wall like most people attempting significant life changes. How the nutritionist responds may make or break Jerry's commitment. A response that minimizes, agrees, denies, blames, avoids, or takes responsibility will serve to diminish Jerry's resolve. Real support takes the form of acknowledging Jerry's feelings without rescuing him.

The nutritionist may respond supportively, "Jerry, I hear you're feeling discouraged and blaming yourself for this recent setback. Let's talk about what needs to happen in order for you to move forward."

This form of communication is called a mirroring response. Like a mirror, it reflects back to the speaker what the respondent has heard the speaker say. Unlike a tape-recorded message, it doesn't play back statements verbatim. It captures feelings and thoughts, while reinforcing the client's responsibility for change.

The Whole Message

An effective mirroring response is built through attending to three interrelated components of the speaker's message:

- **Emotions or feelings:** Virtually all interpersonal communications have an emotional element. It may be minor or trivial, as in instances where people are simply exchanging information. For example, the question "What time is it?" seeks information but may also indicate a slight worry or concern about one's schedule.

- **Key words:** Aside from the emotions they express, spoken words also provide key data about the person or the situation. Someone says, "I just got a new job!" This not only tells you the person has a new job but may also imply that the person had an old job.

- **Nonverbal signals:** Body language conveys additional information about attitudes and feelings. Vocal qualities, such as pitch and tone, communicate attitudes about the content or about the speaker. Facial expressions, such as grins or grimaces, also provide data. Body gestures and movements, such as shaking one's head from side to side or clenching one's fists, help us interpret how the speaker is feeling and what attitudes she or he has toward the topic.

When we are rushed or distracted, we may deliberately ignore one or more elements of a person's message. If we don't want to acknowledge what a person is really saying, we might choose, for example, to attend only to their words and to sidestep the message's tone of delivery (responding "Oh that's great! It's so nice to hear you like summer school" to an adolescent's sarcastic comment, "I just love going to school in the summertime!")

Key Point: *A supportive, mirroring response recognizes all three elements of the speaker's message: emotions + key words + nonverbal signals.*

Creating Supportive, Mirroring Communication

Three basic steps can help you create the supportive, mirroring communication you desire (Figure 1.2). First, identify what the different parts of the message are by looking, listening, and feeling.

Second, integrate in your own mind what all this may mean. The challenge is to sort through the pieces of the message, to find those parts that fit together and those that are discrepant, and to capture the essence of the message.

Third, express in your own words the essence of the person's communication. Play back to the speaker those thoughts, feelings, and even contradictory signals you may be picking up.

Figure 1.2

A Guide to Mirroring Communications

"I pulled a leg muscle in class. It's not too bad; I don't think it'll be a problem."

Step 1: Identify
- Underlying feelings or emotions (worry, fear)
- Key words or message (leg muscle injury)
- Nonverbal signals that support or contradict the expressed emotions or content (facial grimace, furrowed brow)

Step 2: Integrate
Emotions + key words + nonverbal signals
(*She's injured and worried. She hopes it's only minor.*)

Step 3: Express
In your own words state how you understand the person's full communication (emotions + key words + nonverbal signals)
(*Tracy, you look a little more worried about that leg than your words seem to be saying.*)

Let's simplify this seemingly impossible task. Consider the following remark by an athlete experiencing a declining performance:

Linda:

"I'm having some real problems these days. I've had unbelievable amounts of schoolwork . . . endless papers, exams, you know, deadlines, deadlines, deadlines. On top of this, my boss wants me to put in extra hours at the bookstore. He really depends on me, but it puts me in a real bind. . . . Oh yeah, then, there's this little problem at home. My father got laid off and my mother is really worried. . . . No wonder my times are off."

This person has a lot going on in her life. Her whole message is quite consistent—she's dealing with a mixture of pressures and worries. A supportive, mirroring response can capture the essence of her entire message in just a few words.

Your Response:

"Linda, you seem to have a lot to manage. My times would be off, too."

Here is an even briefer response.

Alternative Response:

"Linda, that's a lot. . . . I can really see you're stressed."

You don't need to say much (see Figure 1.3). Search for the core or essential message that the other person is sending. Let yourself feel that message for a moment—and then express to the other person what you understand from the communication.

You don't need to be right. If you are uncertain, you can always ask, "Is this what you're saying?" You can check out or validate your perceptions. Communications are often fuzzy. Allow yourself a margin of error, and take a chance. When you are working to understand another person, she or he usually recognizes your effort. As long as you don't respond defensively, the other person will help you along, repeating the message until both of you know you've *captured the spirit.*

Figure 1.3

Some Ways to Get Started
in Mirroring Communications

Here are a few "lead-ins" to a mirroring response:

"You seem to be saying . . ."
"What I'm hearing is . . ."
"The message I'm getting out of all this is . . ."
"Let me check out what I'm hearing from you . . ."
"Can I tell you what I'm understanding from all this?"
"Are you telling me that . . ."

A REFLECTIVE SUMMARY

Spend some time right now in understanding your own approach to support. It's important that you find your own individual ways of expressing support. Your uniqueness requires that you appreciate how supportive words or expressions would show up in your behavior. To assist you in this process, we have raised some questions for reflection.

- Think about a personal relationship that really supports who you are and where you are going in life. What does support sound like in this relationship? What words most clearly communicate to you that the other person really hears and accepts you?

- Recall a relationship where the responses made to you felt unsupportive, even though the other person thought she or he was being helpful. What did the unsupportive words sound like and how did they make you feel?

- Remember an experience where you gave someone critically needed support. How do you know that person perceived you as being supportive? How did it feel to be supportive? What effects did your support have on the other person?

- Ponder an experience where you wanted to be supportive, but you know your words didn't convey this support to the person. How did you know that what you said wasn't helpful? Did the person become defensive? How did you feel in this situation? What might you have done differently to be perceived as supportive? In retrospect, can you now appreciate the power of your words?

*C*hapter 2

PURPOSE:
THE WHAT, HOW,
AND WHY OF ACTION

*"It isn't that they can't see the solution. It is
that they can't see the problem."*

—G.K. Chesterton

The club was quiet for the moment, like the lull after a battle. Towels draped the equipment. Sweat stains marked the stations of the circuit-training class. Even the rowing machines looked weary from the frenetic energy of the early-bird exercisers. The staff sat back to catch their breath before the onslaught of the noontime crowd.

Just then, the door to the locker room swung wide. A new member charged into the corridor as if leaning into a strong head wind. The majestically rotund man was already breathing heavily, but he headed purposefully toward the cardio room. All morning, Bill had been nervously anticipating his first day at the health club. His doctor had read him the riot act: Exercise or face a possible heart attack. It didn't make it easier for Bill to know that he had at least 50 pounds to shed and that his physical condition seriously interfered with his lovemaking.

He had met Irene, the club manager, the day he signed up 2 weeks ago. Irene had been full of information, but Bill's mind hadn't registered much of what she'd said. He remembered something about the stair climber and $\dot{V}O_2$max and cardiac workouts. Irene's explanations were thorough, but Bill's fears kept him from letting Irene know he couldn't hear.

"Oh yeah, the Stairmaster!" Bill thought as he saw the vast array of machines. "I think I can figure out the buttons. . . . Okay, just step on the pedals here, follow the instructions. Time? Twenty minutes oughta do it. Weight? Two hundred fifty, give or take a little. Level? Oh, 10 is the hardest, so maybe about 8. Bingo! Here we go."

Irene walked by the cardio room minutes after Bill had arrived. The sight she saw could have been a segment from Funniest Home Videos—if it weren't so painful to watch. Here was a seriously overweight 40-year-old, trying to coordinate his movements to those of two little pedals that kept assailing his feet. From the waist up, he looked like a drunk holding onto the railing of a ship in heavy seas.

Irene rushed over to Bill. "Hey, Bill, would you step off for a minute?" she asked in a reassuring voice.

Bill climbed off with an audible sigh of relief. "Yeah, I guess I need to get my feet coordinated," he said apologetically.

"Bill, don't worry about that," Irene responded. "It takes a while to get the hang of it. Besides, I think you were trying to reach your weight-loss goal all in one workout." She smiled reassuringly. "I saw your name on the roster and wanted to come by to say hello. This is your first day, isn't it, Bill?"

"Yeah, it took me a while to get here, but here I am," Bill replied a bit sheepishly.

"Hey, that's great, Bill," Irene said encouragingly. "I remember the program we set up a few weeks ago, so if it's okay with you, I'd like to give you a 5-minute practice session on each of the machines you're going to use in your program. We'll just start slowly today—get used to the machines. You'll like them and you'll get your muscles working. That's doing a lot for your first day."

Bill's whole expression relaxed. "You're the expert," Bill said with appreciation.

"Bill, you get on that Stairmaster, I'll get on this one. We'll go through the setup and get you familiar with some of the levels," Irene coaxed. "After this, we'll do about 5 minutes on the rowing machine and then another 5 on the club's new bikes. How's that sound?"

"Terrific," Bill replied. "It almost sounds as if it could be fun."

Bill had a purpose: He wanted to improve his chances for survival. His plan included working out and losing weight. Irene also had a purpose. She wanted to help Bill achieve his purpose through exercising wisely. Irene was the expert, and she knew Bill might defeat his purpose if he made himself miserable in his workouts or pursued his purpose in an unrealistic manner.

UNDERSTANDING PURPOSE

In the world of health, wellness, and physical activity, people usually offer reasons (or purposes) for the choices they make and the behaviors they engage in. They may express these reasons in words that reflect motives, or we may hear purposes referred to in words that sound like specific goals.

In fitness and health clubs, members may tell you, "I've got to lose 20 pounds," "I want to firm up my muscles," or "I want to be 'heart healthy.' "

Wellness professionals may hear clients cite reasons like "I need to reduce my stress," "I want to have more energy," or "I want to clean up my lifestyle."

In the world of competitive sports, what people say may have a deeper meaning. Individuals may invest a lot of ego in the need to win or perform well. At the professional level, maintaining his or her livelihood may provide an athlete with a strong reason for action.

If you are a hands-on therapist, you may work with people with injuries, disabilities, or body-centered tensions. These people may say the reason for seeing you is to return to activity, to regain as much physical function as possible, or just to become more comfortable in their bodies.

The general term *purpose* encompasses other well-known concepts like goal and motive. If someone says, "I want to be physically active," is that a purpose, a goal, or a motive? Does it matter?

We believe that some distinctions between purpose, goal, and motive will be useful to you in your work.

Purpose Answers the Question "What?"

Purposes relate to a general theme of *what* you want in your life or in a particular experience. They come across as your general intention or desire. Purposes often sound like abstract concepts and may not be easily measured or defined.

A purpose can be general, like a major goal or a broadly defined objective. For example, people talk about such purposes in life as ''being happy,'' ''having financial security,'' or ''being healthy.'' Even though you may think you understand exactly what they mean (because you want to be ''happy'' too), words like happy, healthy, and secure are subject to individual interpretations.

Goal Answers the Question "How?"

Your purpose translated into concrete statements that can be defined, planned, and measured represents your goal. How are you going to become financially secure, happy, or healthy? What specifically are you going to do?

Goals are concrete statements of *how* you are going to achieve your purpose—or how you expect achieving your purpose will look. You may want to be healthy (purpose) and decide to go about it by reducing your consumption of coffee to one cup a day (goal). Or you may want to achieve greater financial security (purpose) by saving $25 a week over the next year (goal). You may want to be happier in your life (purpose) and pursue this by getting a massage each week (goal).

Motive Answers the Question "Why?"

Motives have to do with *why* you want what you want—what needs you want satisfied.

Motives might be thought of as the very subjective and sometimes difficult-to-pinpoint needs underlying your goals and purposes. For instance, you might want to be healthy (purpose) and decide upon a daily aerobics routine (goal). Underlying these decisions could be a need to be independent (motive) so that you don't have to rely on others in your old age.

Or perhaps you want to be happy (purpose) and you plan to train for a marathon (goal). Underlying this purpose and goal is a need for achievement (motive) that drives you toward significant accomplishments.

The Bottom Line of Purpose

In some situations knowing the answers to what, how, and why questions will enable you to work more effectively and to achieve greater success. We're not saying that it's always important to have this information or to be able to distinguish between a purpose, goal, and motive.

We are proposing that you obtain as much information and insight as will be useful to you in helping your clients and athletes reach their goals, achieve their purposes, and satisfy their motivations. The more you know about the people with whom you work, the better able you will be to support them.

Imagine a fitness club member tells you, "I have a goal of losing 15 pounds in 2 months." Do you need to know anything else? We think this could be enough information, yet we also believe learning more about the person might enable you to shape a better program for this client or to help him assess why he's planning to pursue this goal.

Imagine you are a bodyworker with a new client who tells you, "I made a New Year's resolution to get a massage every week" (statement of goal). You could just leave the communication at that, or you could look for answers to all three questions of what, how, and why. Perhaps you could probe or say something like "I'd like to hear what motivated this decision" or "Can you tell me how you came to this resolution?" This client may then tell you she has a lot of neck tension. You could end it here knowing that you need to focus on the neck. Or you could ask another question such as, "Is this the result of an injury or is it a chronic problem?" The answer will guide you to the next question. Your inquiries may reveal external or internal factors contributing to the problem. As a result, your work with this person might include stress reduction techniques, postural suggestions, or even situational solutions (e.g., a telephone headset for someone who spends extensive time on the phone each day).

If, in the moment, you find it awkward or inappropriate to ask another question, make notes of what you know and don't know, and look for opportunities to learn further information later on.

Key Point: *The more ways you can connect people to their purposes, goals, and motives, the greater chances they will have for experiencing success in their endeavors.*

WHAT'S YOUR PURPOSE?

Self-understanding is important for all of us, especially when we want to embark on some new course of action or to reevaluate how we are presently directing our life's energies. We believe this guide to understanding your purposes in life (see Figure 2.1) will enable you to be more insightful not only in your work with yourself, but also in the work you do with others.

No scoring key or a right or wrong set of responses accompanies these questions. They are your guide to the wide world of purposes in your life. Knowing how many purposes underlie your daily choices and actions will also enable you to acknowledge and to address these purposes in others.

SKILL DEVELOPMENT FOR PURPOSE: ASKING QUESTIONS

Two excellent ways to obtain information from people are to

- ask questions, and
- mirror their responses (see Chapter 1—"Skill Development").

The questioning approach may be best in some situations, but you will want to master the mirroring method of obtaining information for situations where questions might produce defensiveness. We will cover both methods in the following sections.

Closed and Open Questions

This list briefly summarizes the differences between closed and open questions.

Closed questions

- can be answered in a few words,
- close off discussion,
- give the questioner control of the conversation,
- direct the discussion, and
- limit the kind of information obtained.

Some examples are

- "How old are you?"
- "Do you like weight training?" and
- "Have you ever had a massage?"

We ask closed questions to obtain facts, clarify information, gain focus, or narrow the area of discussion. Closed questions are essential in information gathering, but they are often overused. Because closed questions

Figure 2.1

A Self-Analysis

How concerned are you about

	Very	Somewhat	Not very
1. Looking good?	❏	❏	❏
2. Being healthy?	❏	❏	❏
3. Feeling sexy?	❏	❏	❏
4. Staying young?	❏	❏	❏
5. Having fun?	❏	❏	❏
6. Setting goals and achieving them?	❏	❏	❏
7. Being the best in competition?	❏	❏	❏
8. Managing your moods?	❏	❏	❏
9. Controlling your tension?	❏	❏	❏
10. Discovering new dimensions of yourself?	❏	❏	❏
11. Learning how to be self-disciplined?	❏	❏	❏
12. Becoming more assertive?	❏	❏	❏
13. Feeling good about yourself?	❏	❏	❏
14. Maintaining an ideal weight?	❏	❏	❏
15. Developing a muscular body?	❏	❏	❏
16. Being with others in a social way?	❏	❏	❏
17. Having time alone?	❏	❏	❏
18. Having a safe outlet for emotions?	❏	❏	❏
19. Feeling competent in what you do?	❏	❏	❏
20. Learning new things about yourself?	❏	❏	❏
21. Developing new skills?	❏	❏	❏

Any others?

attempt to limit the person's response to a few words, they may serve to curtail conversation.

Open questions

- invite a free-flowing answer,
- open up conversations,
- allow the respondent more control of the conversation, and
- usually start with words like how, what, why, could, or would.

Some examples are

- "Would you tell me about your goals?"
- "How do you think you can best improve your health?" and
- "What would you like to get out of our session today?"

An open question requires an explanation and invites discussion. When you are trying to understand another person's perspective or way of viewing the world, it's advisable to invite remarks without the structure imposed by closed questions.

Choosing One Type of Question Over the Other

Time is a critical factor in determining which kind of question you ask. When you don't have a lot of time, you may need to ask direct, closed questions that tell you exactly what you need to know. Open questions allow speakers to talk at whatever length they choose. When you can't afford the time, don't invite a lengthy response.

Look at how the same issue gets dealt with through a closed, compared with an open, question.

Closed Question	Open Question
Do you like running?	What sports do you like?
Are you feeling tired?	How are you feeling?
Do you want to lose weight?	What are your goals?
You agree with me, don't you?	What's your opinion?
Do you want to train at 9:00 a.m. on Tuesday?	What schedule suits you best?

One type of question is not necessarily better than the other; each has its value. To decide which type to use, be clear about what information you need and what kind of question best suits the situation.

Key Point: *If you need to limit or control the discussion, use closed questions. If you want someone to explore an issue, use open questions.*

Three Questions About the Question You're Asking

When you are preparing questions for an interview or for ongoing use in your professional work, you may want to run your potential questions through the filters of the following three questions.

What Do You Need to Know?   Before you start asking questions, you will want to be very clear about what it is you want to know.

Will the Question You Ask Get the Information You Need?   If you want to know about a person's attitudes toward competition, you need to ask the right question. A direct question like "How do you feel about competitive sports and games?" might work better than an indirect question like "Do you like tennis [a competitive game]?"

How Will Your Question Impact Your Respondent?   You might ask someone "Would you tell me why losing 20 pounds is so important to you?" but the question could possibly offend the person or be interpreted as intrusive. Either reaction to the question stands a chance of sealing off communication. Sometimes you would like to ask a justifiable question, but the relationship isn't ready for it. When this is the case, it's probably best to keep track of the information you have and the information you still need. The right time to ask the right question will come.

Common Problems in Asking Questions

Asking a good question is an art. It takes practice learning how to be clear about what you need to know and how to translate that need into a question that someone else understands and is willing to answer.

Some common pitfalls occur in asking questions. Check yourself to be sure you aren't falling into one of these traps.

Asking Double-Barreled Questions.   This is an error of asking two questions at the same time. It may confuse the respondent and can make the respondent's task more complex. Further, if both questions are important, you may get diluted, low-impact responses by requiring the respondent to answer both at the same time. Here are some examples:

- "What do you need to know about the club, and what sports interest you most?"
- "How much experience have you had with massage? Are you interested in learning yoga?"

- "How motivated are you to regain the full range of movement in your leg, and how did you injure yourself in the first place?"

- "What are you willing to change about your eating habits, and what kinds of problems have you had with eating plans in the past?"

Asking Leading Questions. A leading question is phrased in a way that makes it easier or more tempting for the interviewee to answer in a particular way. This creates biased responses or answers because you indirectly tell the respondent what the supposed right ones are. Here are some examples:

- "Wouldn't you like to try this machine?"

- "With your level of stress, don't you think you ought to get a weekly massage?"

- "Wouldn't it be better if you started your physio more gradually?"

- "Don't you think with all that weight you're carrying you ought to stop eating those donuts?"

Asking Bipolar Questions. A bipolar question offers the interviewee only two opposing responses when, in fact, more than two choices exist. In a more subtle way, this form of question biases the respondent by making it seem as if there are no other possible answers. Here are some examples:

- "Do you approve or disapprove of the way I teach the class?"

- "Would you rather take stress management training or enroll in a healthy eating class?"

- "Would you rather come today or tomorrow?"

- "Are you a vegetarian or a meat eater?"

How to Ask Questions Without Asking Questions

In Chapter 1 you learned about mirroring communications. This technique has many interesting applications, including its use in drawing out information. By mirroring a speaker's remarks, you encourage her or him to continue talking while allowing the speaker control of the direction of the conversation. This has clear advantages:

- It allows the speaker to feel in control.

- It reduces the speaker's defensiveness.

- It permits the speaker to follow her agenda, rather than one you dictate.

- It keeps your intentional or unintentional biases to a minimum.

- It slows down the action so you don't jump to conclusions.

Examine the following interview between a personal trainer and a new client. Notice how a mirroring response draws out information from the client.

Trainer: "Jean, would you tell me what you'd like to get out of an exercise program?" [Open question]

Jean: "Well, I want to lose a few pounds and shape up."

Trainer: "Okay, so you'd like to lose weight and firm up." [Mirroring response]

Jean: "Yeah, I could stand to lose about 15 pounds and I don't just want to diet. I'd like to have some muscles that I can flex."

Trainer: "So, you want to be stronger and more muscular looking [?]" [Mirroring response]

Jean: "That's right. I'm tired of looking so dumpy and feeling dumpy, too. I think I'd like myself better if I looked better in my clothes."

Trainer: "I see. You're hoping to feel better about yourself by getting fit." [Mirroring response]

Jean: "Well, I don't expect to change overnight and I'm not expecting miracles, but I would like eventually to fit into a size-8 dress and feel sexier."

Trainer: "Jean, what do you think it'll take to reach these goals?" [Open question]

Jean: "I'm not sure. You're the expert on that . . . but I was hoping that I could make some progress by the time I go to Club Med next month."

Trainer: "Some progress by next month [?]" [Mirroring response with an emphasis on the word some]

Jean: "Well, you know, if I work out with you every day, I should be able to lose some weight in a month's time. Of course, I'll cut back on eating, too."

Trainer: "So, your plan is to work out daily and cut back on eating." [Mirroring response]

Jean: "Yeah . . . I don't expect to lose it all, maybe about 5 pounds. Does that sound reasonable?"

The trainer used a combination of open questions and mirroring responses. The trainer's mirroring responses informed Jean that the trainer understood what she had said and gave her an opportunity to modify or clarify her comments.

The conversation had a unique quality: Even though Jean may have been hoping she could lose 15 pounds in a month, part of her knew it was unrealistic. If the trainer had told her this at the very beginning, Jean might have had a negative reaction. By mirroring Jean's comments, the trainer gave Jean an opportunity to reflect realistically on her request. In the end, she came to her own conclusion that "maybe about 5 pounds" was a more realistic goal for the first month.

The trainer refrained from jumping in with a plan too quickly. She could have stopped after the first sentence when Jean told her she wanted to lose a few pounds and firm up. Instead, by being supportive, by mirroring Jean's thoughts and feelings, the trainer guided her to be more explicit—and realistic—about her goals and motives, ensuring a reasonable chance for her to be successful.

SKILL DEVELOPMENT FOR PURPOSE: INTERVIEWING

An interview is an interaction between two or more people, in which one person assumes the role of questioner. The interviewer is expected to set the agenda and direct the conversation. Someone who comes to you for information will assume the role of interviewer. When you want information from someone, you take on the interviewer's role.

The roles of interviewer and interviewee may switch back and forth. If you are applying for a job, you will typically be in the role of the interviewee. If you need information about the organization you are applying to, you take on the role of interviewer. An interaction between a health/fitness professional and a client often looks like a relationship in which two people alternately ask and answer questions. Sometimes one person is the interviewer and the other the interviewee; then the roles switch.

Role, Resources, and Situation (RRS) as Guides to Interviewing

We discussed the importance of the RRS formula in the previous chapter. Let's see how Role, Resources, and Situational considerations play into an interview plan.

What's Your Role?

Knowing your role helps you determine the legitimacy of your questions. It sets limits to the kinds of questions you can ask your students, clients, or athletes. For example, an exercise psychologist doing a research project may be able to ask all kinds of questions about how exercise impacts people's private lives; yet a personal trainer working with individuals has certain professional constraints on the kinds of questions permissible to ask her or his clients.

What do you think are the boundaries of questions you can legitimately ask in your role as a health/fitness professional?

What Are Your Resources?

Being aware of what you can do with the information you gather and how much time you have available for inquiry serves as a guide to the design of an interview that is reasonable for you. For example, how fruitful would it be to ask if a person likes swimming when there are no pools available? Or, if you only have 10 minutes to gather information, what questions will give you the best information in the time available?

What's the Situation?

Aspects of the situation may further define the questions you can ask, when you can ask them, and where would be the best place to ask them. For example, personal questions are best asked in a place that allows privacy. Asking questions when someone is in a rush to get back to work will reduce the amount and validity of the information you obtain. Strive to create a time and place that are most conducive to the nature of the interview you have planned.

Interviews Have Structure—More or Less

On many occasions the information you need is confined to a limited area. As a physiotherapist, you may want to know how well your clients are following your prescriptions. If you are a coach, you may want to find out how different players respond to your style of coaching. Personal trainers may want to know if clients' original goals have changed. As a high school teacher, you may want to identify the place sports and exercise occupy in students' lives.

You will find it useful to follow this 8-step process when planning your interviews (see Figure 2.2):

Step 1. State your overall purpose. The clearer you can be about your purpose for the interview, the easier it will be to develop the right questions.

Step 2. Define your specific needs. Your purpose can be translated into specific statements of what you want to know. If you are interested in feedback about how well the injured athletes are following your pre-scriptions, you might translate this general purpose into statements like

"I want to know . . .

. . . if my instructions were clear."

. . . if they remember my prescriptions."

. . . if they thought my prescriptions were doable."

. . . how successful they were in carrying out the prescriptions."

. . . how successful they felt the prescriptions were in improving their conditions."

Step 3. Form your questions. Let's take the first statement above:

"I want to know if my instructions were clear."

Consider the following questions you might ask to elicit that information:

"How clear have my instructions been about at-home work?"

"Were my instructions clear?"

"You found my instructions clear, didn't you?"

"What kinds of problems do you have following my instructions?"

"Do you understand my instructions and are you always able to follow them?"

Step 4. Critique your questions. Of the five questions listed above, the first two would probably be most helpful in getting you the information you need without leading or confusing your interviewee.

"How clear have my instructions been about at-home work?" is specific and focused on the issue.

"Were my instructions clear?" will work only if you have previously defined which instructions you're talking about.

"You found my instructions clear, didn't you?" is a leading question that tells the respondent what answer you want.

"What kinds of problems do you have following my instructions?" is also a leading question in that it presumes the person has had problems with your instructions.

"Do you understand my instructions and are you always able to follow them?" is a double-barreled question—you've asked two questions at the same time. Your respondent may be confused about which one to answer first or may forget one of the questions.

Step 5. Determine a logical arrangement. Imagine you are a lifestyle management consultant and you are interviewing a new client. You have come up with the following questions:

"What kind of schedule would best suit you?"

"What would you like to get out of this program?"

"What do I need to know about you so I can be most effective in my work with you?"

"What would you like to know about me?"

"What experiences with making lifestyle changes have you had in the past?"

"What brings you to this decision to work with me?"

If you were to ask these questions, you would surely want to arrange them in a different order. Although other arrangements may make sense, this sequence seems to have a logical flow:

1. "What brings you to this decision to work with me?"

2. "What experiences with making lifestyle changes have you had in the past?"

3. "What would you like to get out of this program?"

4. "What do I need to know about you so I can be most effective in my work with you?"

5. "What would you like to know about me?"

6. "What kind of schedule would best suit you?"

Notice how the questions flow from one another, with each question setting the stage for the next question. For example, by asking the person about prior experiences in making lifestyle changes, you prepare the interviewee for a question about present goals.

Step 6. Conduct a trial test. Even though the questions may make perfect sense to you, your expert knowledge may create blind spots about your topic. You need to ask these questions of a few people who are like the people you eventually intend to interview. Not only would you ask them the questions as if you were conducting a real interview, but following the interview you would also review the questions with your interviewees to get additional feedback about your questions and the order in which you asked them.

Step 7. Modify your questions. The feedback from your trial sample might cause you to rephrase some of your questions, to add some new ones, or to adjust the order.

Step 8. Interview your client. Now you can conduct your interview with assurance that you are using questions that will get you the information you need. Make sure that the conditions under which you interview are conducive to getting the best answers.

Figure 2.2

Checklist for Developing an Interview

_____ 1. Overall purpose: Write down your general purpose.

_____ 2. Specific needs: Translate your purpose into specific statements of what you want to know.

_____ 3. Form questions: Turn the specific statements into questions, using the simplest language possible.

_____ 4. Critique questions: Check for faulty question structure (leading, double-barreled, bipolar).

_____ 5. Logical arrangement: Arrange questions in an order that makes sense to you and that will make sense to the interviewee.

_____ 6. Trial test: Ask the questions to a few people who are like the people you want to interview. Get feedback on the questions and review the answers to determine if they are telling you what you want to know.

_____ 7. Modify: Modify your questions based on the feedback.

_____ 8. Interview your client: Put your questions into action at the right time and place.

A REFLECTIVE SUMMARY

Implicit in the concept of support is a sense of purpose. Toward what ends are we supporting another person?

There is a fable about a young man standing by a roadside watching an old man dig a hole. After a while the bystander asked the old man if he could help him shovel the hole. The man looked up, smiled appreciatively, and without words tossed the young man a shovel. Hours went by before the work was done. The two sweat-drenched men paused and took a long drink of water from a cool pitcher sitting in the shade. The young bystander shook hands with the old man and began to walk away. After a few steps, he turned back to give a final wave only to see that the old man was now shoveling dirt back into the hole. He ran up to the man and exclaimed in exasperation, "What are you doing? I thought you were trying to dig a hole!" The old man smiled benignly and said, "I was. Now I'm filling it back up."

As farfetched as this fable may seem, we believe this story about a young man who assists in a task without understanding its point teaches an important lesson. Support needs to be understood in the context of purpose, and that purpose is most fully answered by examining the questions of what people want, why they want it, and how they plan to attain it. We often hear people respond to such questions as "Why did you climb that mountain?" with facile answers like "Because it's there!" This kind of vague answer may have a certain mystique, but professionals need to ask at least one further question, such as "Would you please tell me more?"

In our own lives, we may pursue paths because of motivations that are only partially revealed to us. Midlife comes and we discover that indeed the path we have trod for the past two or three decades really belonged to someone else or perhaps poorly suited our deeply wished-for ends.

We encourage you not only to consider the whats, whys, and hows of your own actions, but also to gather information from the people with whom you work so that you can help them reach their goals more efficiently and successfully.

Chapter 3

INTEGRITY:
ESTABLISHING PERSONAL
AND PROFESSIONAL BOUNDARIES

"There is dignity in work only when it is work freely accepted."

—Albert Camus

Bobby had been up for about half an hour and was just finishing his morning stretch routine when the call came through. He picked up the phone on the second ring. It was Harvey, his 7:00 a.m. appointment. "Bobby," he said, "I'm sorry. I have to cancel out on you this morning."

Bobby's face showed concern. "Are you all right, Harvey?"

"Yeah, I'm fine, Bobby," he responded. "It's just that I have to take an out-of-town client for breakfast."

Bobby relaxed and replied, "Great, so we'll meet on Friday as scheduled . . . and I'd like to be clear that you'll be charged $25 according to our agreement on cancellations."

Harvey said, "That's fine with me. This wasn't an emergency."

Bobby reflected on how smoothly this transaction went, and how long he had struggled to establish this policy. More than a year ago he realized he was doing no one a favor by not charging for cancellations. He felt resentment, and his devaluing of his own time only served to reinforce his clients' lack of commitment.

After making a few calls and catching up on some bookkeeping, Bobby left to meet his 9:00 a.m. client at the gym. He felt a bit apprehensive knowing that it was time to confront Erica. It had become all too clear that her goal to seduce him was greater than her desire to work out. Each session he thought he had established his boundaries in regard to the personal side of training, yet she persisted in her attempts to go beyond those limits. Bobby knew he had to be direct, unequivocal, and willing to lose her as his client.

Erica's greeting reinforced his concern. She walked up to him in the aerobics room and kissed him slowly on the cheek.

Bobby stepped back and, looking Erica straight in the eyes, spoke in a calm, yet strong voice. "Erica, good morning. I need to discuss this training relationship before we go any further. . . ."

Erica cut him off in midsentence. "Oh, come on Bobby, let's not get into that again. I hate it when you get so serious."

Bobby knew in that moment that her side of the relationship was not up for discussion. It was a struggle to keep Erica's interactions within bounds, especially when her primary interest was in him and not in her training. "Erica, I appreciate that you would like this relationship to be different from what it is, yet I have been clear before and I want to be clear now that these are not the terms of my agreement with you."

Erica looked surprised, "Hey, Bobby, I thought you were interested. . . . I guess I misread you."

Without the slightest reproach in his voice, Bobby replied, "I'm sorry, Erica. . . . I'm sorry if I was misleading in any way. Why don't we take it from here? I would be glad to continue working together as long as we have this issue completely clear between us. I do not get romantically involved with my clients—in or out of the gym."

Erica was silent for a long moment before responding, "I'm disappointed, but I do like training with you, Bobby, so I'll agree to your terms. Let's get started."

"Sounds good to me," Bobby said with an inward sigh of relief.

What do we mean by the term *boundaries*? A tennis court has boundaries. So does a football field, a basketball court, and a swimming pool. Boundaries allow you to determine when the football goes between the goalposts, when a swimmer is in the right lane, or when a basketball player is out-of-bounds. As a health/fitness professional, you need boundaries for the same reason a playing field needs them. They serve as guides for deciding what is within limits and what is out-of-bounds.

In sports as in life, action is governed by the added element of the rules of the game. Sometimes these rules are clear, like "Stopping at red lights." Other times, rules require an element of interpretation. We see this quite vividly when referees huddle to make judgment calls about whether actions were intentional or accidental.

You may wonder about Bobby's judgment calls in the opening story. He asked Harvey whether he was "all right" to determine whether his cancellation policy would apply. If Harvey had been sick, Bobby might not have charged the $25 fee. You may have found yourself agreeing with Bobby's response to Erica, and you may personally avoid mixing business with pleasure. Yet, it might be hard to find clearly drawn professional boundaries between yourself and your clients.

In this chapter the interpretation of integrity as a matter of setting and respecting boundaries encompasses far more than drawing lines on playing fields. A subjective element is often present in establishing boundaries— and over time, our subjective views may change.

The more effort you invest in clarifying your rules and boundaries, the more "Out-of-bounds!" indicates an alert rather than a crisis. Your integrity derives not only from adherence to the rules of your profession but also from an awareness of your personal boundaries for engaging life.

PROFESSIONAL BOUNDARIES

Professional boundaries stem from definitions of your role, job skills, and responsibilities. The longer a profession has been in existence, the more likely it is to be governed by professional associations that delimit actions considered fair or foul. Most professions have some equivalent of an ethical review board to debate the inevitable gray areas that emerge in practice. Professions are not static entities, but rather dynamic, evolving systems that must continually examine and monitor the frontiers of practice. Current professional boundaries may help guide your actions in a wide array of situations, but they will never cover all events you are likely to encounter in your career.

One way we develop professional boundaries is through observation and imitation. During our training, we watch others, we receive supervision, and we are exposed to different kinds of instruction. We may take courses on communication, leadership, psychology, and business. As we learn the how-tos of our jobs, we also develop a sense of the interpersonal boundaries of our work. Our teachers, supervisors, and mentors reveal to us in direct and indirect ways what professional means. In many of our chosen professions, we undertake specific training and certification that are usually accompanied by their own explicit professional codes.

There may still be some gray areas for you. To help you sort through the different messages you may have been exposed to during your professional development, we ask you to take some time to complete the exercise in Figure 3.1. As you reflect on the opening words of the sentences in this exercise, let your mind fill in the blanks with what you believe to be the different rules or boundaries you have understood about your professional role. Make notes on your reflections in the spaces provided.

What do these notes tell you about your professional boundaries? How do you feel about what you have written? What do you think you should keep? What would you like to change? Why? What might you do to clear up some of the conflicting messages appearing in your answers?

PERSONAL BOUNDARIES

Personal boundaries represent your deep values and beliefs. Although they may mirror public morality or principles in society and religion, ultimately they are yours. Personal boundaries delineate where your self lives and how you construe your personal role and responsibilities in the world. Partly, they're statements of "This is me!" or "This is not me!" Boundaries may also be thought of as descriptors of your personal code of conduct. You use these values and beliefs to make decisions about what behaviors are appropriate and inappropriate for yourself and others. They are your guides, especially in the gray areas of life.

The development of personal boundaries is a lifelong process. Experiences in childhood may shape some of your beliefs, values, and even your self-definitions. Some of these messages push you forward, others may hold you back. Yet, you are not a fixed entity. You continue to have new experiences and to learn new ideas. Exposure to new situations may serve to broaden your concepts about life or to reaffirm previously held values. Feedback from others and personal reflection can also help you understand your boundaries.

Personal boundaries live in your heart—past all the "shoulds" and "shouldn'ts." Integrity, then, is a felt sense of deep personal acceptance. From this personal acceptance, your truth emerges to answer questions of conduct.

Figure 3.1

Statements to Lead You to Your Boundaries

Write down your responses to the following statements:

"You should always . . ."

"You should never . . ."

"The way to be successful is to . . ."

"In working with my clients/athletes, it is my business to . . ."

"In working with my clients/athletes, it is none of my business to . . ."

"A good rule of thumb is . . ."

GUIDELINES FOR DEVELOPING BOUNDARIES

We suggest you consider four guidelines—respect, understanding, caring, and fairness—in developing your boundaries. We offer these to clarify and simplify an ever-present philosophical debate about the self in relationship to others.

- **Respect:** Do you feel a clear sense of respect for yourself in the things you do and in the way you live your life? Do you believe others experience a respectful attitude in your behavior toward them?

- **Understanding:** Do you treat yourself with understanding and acceptance? Or are you quick to blame yourself or to find fault? Do you appreciate the dilemmas in your life, the difficulties of the decisions you must make, and the fact of your humanity? Do you express understanding and acceptance to others?

- **Caring:** Are you careful with yourself, avoiding situations and activities that would jeopardize you physically or emotionally? Are you careful with others, making sure nothing you do will cause them physical or emotional harm?

- **Fairness:** Are you equitable in the ways you balance your needs and the needs of others? Do you operate with double standards or are you consistent? Are you clear in your agreements and commitments?

An Opportunity for Reflection

The questions in Figure 3.2 provide an opportunity to examine yourself according to the four guidelines for developing boundaries. Whatever your answers, we encourage you to treat yourself with respect, understanding, caring, and fairness, even while you complete this self-reflection exercise.

There's no answer key for this exercise. It is meant as a mirror of your behaviors and those you create with others. You may notice that your answers for personal relationships differ from those for professional ones. If so, what sense do you make of this?

Several times you may have answered, Well, sometimes I do that, and sometimes I don't. It's important to check out those ''sometimes'' to better understand conditions that influence your actions.

How comfortable are you with your answers? Do they provide direction for making desirable changes in how you relate to yourself and to others? What small step toward change can you take today?

Figure 3.2

A Self-Reflection on Boundaries in Professional and Personal Relationships

Consider the following questions. Make notes as you go through them to assist your process of reflection.

1. Do I make myself responsible for another person's happiness?
2. Do I put others in the position of being responsible for my happiness?
3. Do I take on the job of providing another person's self-esteem?
4. Do I rely on others to give me positive feelings of self-esteem?
5. Do I deny my own feelings so someone else can feel good?
6. Do I ignore others' feelings to make myself feel good?
7. Do I allow myself to be used as a dumping ground for another person's bad feelings?
8. Do I dump my feelings on others?
9. Do I feel physically and emotionally safe in situations I put myself in?
10. Do I put others in physical or emotional jeopardy?
11. Do I respect my body's needs and limits?
12. Do I respect others' bodily needs and limits?
13. Do I accept all parts of myself, even the ones that I want to improve?
14. Do I feel accepting and noncritical of others while they are in the process of change?

Plugging Boundaries Into the RRS Formula

The RRS formula comes into play as a further means for clarifying personal and professional boundaries. Here's how role, resources, and situational considerations may apply.

Role

Maybe you work in a job where the rules of conduct are posted on the wall. Or say you have a boss who tells you exactly what you can and can't do. It's also possible that you belong to a professional group that requires adherence to a code of conduct.

Maybe it's less clear than this. Your job may be such that at times you feel you have to wing it. Even when rules are posted and a boss is explicit and the job is well defined, judgment calls have to be made. The more professional a job is, the more gray areas it seems to present. And the more gray areas you encounter in your work, the more you will need to check your decisions against your personal boundaries.

For example, if there are no professional rules about charging clients for canceled sessions, you may need to rely on your personal values for guidance. What do you need in this situation to feel respectful, understanding, caring, and fair, toward both yourself and your client? The decisions you make come to represent your personal and professional boundaries.

Resources

What are your personal and professional resources? You have certain talents and skills, and you have been educated and trained in your field. And you have time—which is limited.

Besides yourself, what other resources are available to you? You may be part of a network of professionals or connected to resources that expand your possibilities for information, support, and referral. If you are affiliated with a school, clinic, club, or hospital, you can plug into these systems.

How much of your personal resources you commit to your professional role is an individual decision. How far beyond the call of duty will you reach?

Your levels of involvement might be guided by your answers to the questions of what respect, understanding, caring, and fairness look like in specific situations. Agreements you have made with others will greatly assist you in keeping clear about resource boundaries. When a client requests exceptions, additions, or straight-out changes to your practice, boundaries established in previous agreements will serve as your guide.

If you devote too many of your personal resources to your work, you could burn out. For a while, you might get away with overextending yourself, but over months and years, it can take its toll. It's good to be clear about how much you need to hold in reserve for yourself.

An Exercise in Time.   One measure of commitment is time. How much time do you make available for work, for family, for career pursuits, and for yourself?

Try the exercise in Figure 3.3. Imagine a typical day during your work week. Apportion the time you would ideally like to spend on various activities. Then look at your real life. How much time do you actually spend on these activities? What do the discrepancies between the real and the ideal tell you about how you are managing one of your most important personal resources—time?

Having clear boundaries around your personal resources allows you to make good decisions about the responsibilities you take on. Most people are amazed when they compare all their commitments to the hours they actually have available. Is there any wonder that stress disorders are considered a modern-day epidemic?

Situation

The last element in the RRS formula is the situation itself. Let's go back to Bobby's decisions regarding Harvey's cancellation and Erica's romantic intentions. Bobby considered the situations—allowing for exceptions—and then made his decisions based on his agreements and boundaries. Had Harvey been sick or confronted with an emergency, the situation would have altered Bobby's decision. Had he allowed for romance in his work, it would have been reflected in his responses to Erica.

Sometimes your best guide is how a situation feels in your heart. At times you may be asked to do things that fall within your role and that require resources which you have, but the actions just don't feel right. What is being asked for, directly or indirectly, may be a violation of your sense of yourself—your integrity.

These situations may occur because others do not perceive your boundaries in the same way that you do. The following scenarios may illustrate the issue:

- A high school student in an education class asks your permission to turn in a report 1 week late. The reason he gives is that he is scheduled to compete in a national-level tennis tournament.

- A talented swimmer repeatedly misses practice, yet continues to improve on her swimming times. You have suspended her from the team because she has missed one too many practices. She asks you to reconsider, offering valid arguments that her performance continues to improve and that the team won't do as well without her.

- A health club member continually seeks your advice on what workout he should do, which instructors will be best for him, and how long he should exercise to achieve various results. He now wants your opinion about whether he should work out in the morning or in the evening. You tell him about physiological differences reported in research, but he presses you to make an expert decision for him.

Figure 3.3

Resources: Your *Ideal* Versus *Real* Time Distribution

Using a 24-hour day, make two estimates of time for each category below:

- First, estimate the number of hours you would *ideally* like to spend on this category of activity.
- Second, estimate the actual amount of time you devote to it.

After doing this, consider the meaning of the differences between your ideal and your real time investments.

Activity	Your Ideal Time	Your Actual Time
Work	_____	_____
Study	_____	_____
Exercise	_____	_____
Meals	_____	_____
Recreation	_____	_____
Sleep	_____	_____
Personal hygiene	_____	_____
Travel	_____	_____
Shopping	_____	_____
Chores	_____	_____
Family	_____	_____
Friends	_____	_____
Intimate relations	_____	_____
Spiritual activities	_____	_____
Other activities	_____	_____
	_____	_____
Total hours	_____	_____

What conclusions might you draw from this analysis?

_____

_____

_____

_____

There is no right answer to any of these scenarios. Your response depends on values that you carry deep within yourself. You may believe that fairness requires that you adhere to an unalterable due date for the high school student; that swimming isn't about winning, it's about reliability and teamwork; or that the club member's dependency on you is unacceptable. Only you can make these subtle distinctions as you define boundaries around your self.

You may have had a hard time answering the requests made in the preceding three scenarios because you didn't know all aspects of the situation.

- The tennis player may have been totally surprised by his own success in regional competition.

- The swimmer may have been juggling family responsibilities for younger siblings with school and sports.

- The dependent health club member may have recently come back from coronary bypass surgery and been terribly frightened about doing something wrong.

Exceptions to rules may be justified by unusual out-of-the-ordinary circumstances. If you find yourself making so many exceptions that living by the rule becomes the exception, you may want to examine what criteria for exceptional circumstances you have or what kind of situation you are in.

Boundary Review

The definitions of many roles evolve over time. What is a mother's or a father's role? Is a high school teacher supposed to teach or discipline? How much does a bodyworker need to know about a client's personal life? What are your responsibilities as a fitness leader? Unless you are working in a narrowly defined, contractual job, you will typically be asked to make judgment calls.

Remembering the guidelines of role, resources, and situation will help you navigate these murky waters. The formula will also help you understand how to reach satisfactory agreements with others, the subject of our next Skill Development section.

Key Point: *If we respect the limits of our personal resources, it will be far easier to know the boundaries of our roles.*

SKILL DEVELOPMENT FOR INTEGRITY: AGREEMENTS AND CONTRACTS

A health club member signs a contract when joining a club. A student enters into a learning contract in a stress management course. A personal trainer makes an agreement with a client about schedules and payments. A physiotherapy patient consents to three visits per week for 2 months. A nutritionist agrees to work for a salary at a clinic. A college student on athletic scholarship signs a contract with her school.

An agreement may be defined as "an arrangement as to a course of action," while a contract may be defined as a binding agreement that usually involves legal consequences if the terms of the contract are broken.

Agreements and contracts are about boundaries, about who does what, when, where, how, and under what terms. Some agreements are implicit or assumed; others are explicit and clear. The terms of some contracts might be ambiguous, allowing room for different interpretations. Other contracts are definite, with terms that spell out exactly what is expected.

Assumed Agreements

The fewer assumptions we make in our agreements with others, the better off we all will be. Even if you are operating in good faith, you may have assumptions about your agreement that are different from those the other person holds.

Let's look at a few situations in which assumed agreements may develop.

- Imagine an aerobics class where some participants go into free-style dance and clash with the leader. If the leader does nothing to correct the situation, the assumed agreement is that you can do what you want in this class.

- What happens if your client continually shows up late for your 1-hour bodywork session, yet you always give him a full hour? Your client may assume your agreement is that he is entitled to a full hour no matter when he shows up.

- Imagine your club has a 20-minute limit on the cardio machines during peak hours, yet a member stays on a machine for 45 minutes every evening at 6:00 p.m. 5 days in a row. She may be assuming that (a) the rule doesn't apply to her, (b) the rule isn't really a rule, or (c) 6:00 p.m. isn't a peak hour.

- If a team has a rule about traveling to out-of-town games on the school bus, but seniors usually take their own cars, it may be assumed that seniors have an agreement exempting them from the rule.

All these situations have one thing in common: People observe behavior patterns and infer the rules or boundaries.

Regardless of the stated rule or agreement, actions speak louder than words. Each time a boundary infraction occurs without comment or penalty, it may alter the boundary. In time, everyone may believe the rule has changed.

If a coach is always 10 minutes late for practice, 10 after the hour becomes the assumed agreed-upon time for the start of practice. If the coach tries to change her behavior, she will find it difficult to counter what has become the norm.

The Psychological Contract

Assumed agreements make up part of what is known as the psychological contract. Your personal history causes you to develop expectations of others' behaviors. It's your birthday and you assume that everyone will make a fuss. You get a new job and assume you will be rewarded for good work. You enter a new relationship and assume because you give a lot, the other person will also. You make doctors' appointments and expect you will be kept waiting. You register in university courses and expect Catch 22s or administrative snares. You go to work and expect to be told what to do. Whatever your experience, you have expectations! They may be expectations of fair and respectful treatment or of indifferent and impersonal behavior.

As a health/fitness professional, you have expectations of the people with whom you work, and they have expectations of you. You may know what you expect of yourself, but be less sure about what others expect from you. Without complete information you may mistakenly assume you know what is expected of you and operate on these assumptions.

Being successful in your job involves *initiating* conversations to make explicit any expectations others have of you, as well as yours of them. Such dialogs will allow you to know exactly in which areas you should put your energy and in which areas you are accountable.

Key Point: *When in doubt, check it out. Ask what someone expects of you.*

Terms of Agreement

A useful way to think about the terms of your agreement with another person is to examine it in the light of the questions: Who? What? When? Where? and How?

Who is involved? Is it you and an athlete? You and a client? Part of the who question refers to your respective roles. Is your client a minor who requires parental consent to participate in the program? Does your client have known health risks? Have appropriate groups licensed or certified you to do your job?

What is involved, or what is your agreement about? What are your and the other person's purposes? Are you providing a service? What are you expected to do to achieve your purpose? What is the other person expected to do? Do some purposes seem so obvious that you assume them instead of making them explicit?

When does the agreed-to activity happen? It's important to know when certain things are expected to happen, and also for how long or over what period of time. If a client hired you for 2 hours a week, you might want to stipulate not only the exact hours of meeting but also the minimal duration of your contract, for example, 6 weeks. Another critical aspect of this question is when does your agreement not apply. You may encounter

---

Figure 3.4

Who, What, When, Where, and How

- **Who is involved?** What are their roles? What are their distinguishing features (*job, age, health, ability*)?
- **What is involved?** What is the agreement about? What are you doing? What is the other person to do? Who is responsible for what?
- **When does this happen?** How often, how long, and over what period of time? And when doesn't this happen? What are the limits?
- **Where does this happen?** What place? What conditions? And where doesn't it happen? What places are inappropriate?
- **How does this happen?** What are the methods? What is your style? What methods are excluded? What will you NOT do?

clients during off hours when your clients may want to discuss their particular situation with you. Is this part of your agreement? Is this occasion another "when" of your agreement?

Where does and doesn't this agreed-upon transaction take place? Do you have an office or a studio? Do you meet to discuss your clients' performance with them in a private setting like their homes or your house? If you meet a client at a party, is it okay to engage in conversation with her about her training program?

How do you carry out this agreement? What does doing it look like? What are its specific goals? What methods are you trained/certified to use and which lie beyond your training or certification? What can you do as a certified athletic therapist? What boundaries does your work as a personal trainer have? How do you work with clients as a bodyworker?

Another aspect of the how question relates to individual style. Some hands-on therapists may do only massage, while others may incorporate stress-reduction techniques. Some personal trainers work out with their clients; others watch and supervise. Making your methods explicit involves discussing your style of working with people.

Formal and Informal Agreements

It's our experience that informal agreements may often break down because one or both parties don't expect the terms to be respected or the agreement does not stipulate any real consequences for failing to meet conditions. Informal agreements give both sides excuses to back out. Two people "informally" agree to study together whenever they can—until one of them fails to show up. A client agrees to try a new fitness approach for a while, to see what happens, but how long is a while?

Referring to an arrangement as an informal agreement may have to do with fear and doubt: fear that a more formal contract would be too binding; doubt that you or the other person will live up to the terms of a real agreement. Informal agreements may be a way of sitting on the fence and not making commitments. That might be just fine for you under the circumstances! However, if it's not, you will want to work toward a formal agreement.

All real agreements are formal because in them you take the time necessary to be explicit about all the expectations of all the parties and all the answers to who, what, when, where, and how. Even when you are uncertain about aspects of your transaction, you can still have a formal agreement that states what you and the other party need (who, what, when, where, and how) to come to more definite terms.

A mistaken notion is that an agreement is informal unless it is written. You can have a verbal formal agreement, but verbal agreements can be problematic because of memory lapses, semantics, or trustworthiness. You may forget the terms. Your idea of paying at the beginning of the month may mean paying before the 15th, while the other party seeks payment within several days of the 1st. You may have no intention of living up to the agreement because as Bart Simpson says, "You can't prove a thing!"

A Guide to Making Agreements

We suggest you use the guide in Figure 3.5 to help you identify elements of your agreements with others. Try applying the guide in discussions with clients, athletes, or students to determine its value for your work, and to help you identify boundaries and agendas in your agreements.

A Final Check on Your Agreements

Imagine you have just finished a discussion with one of your clients, athletes, or students and have reached an agreement about working together. The agreement has been written and signed. You are now reflecting on the meeting and evaluating what has transpired. The following checklist (see Figure 3.6) might be useful in reviewing the process of this discussion and the agreements reached.

A REFLECTIVE SUMMARY

Integrity is about boundaries; about fairness and respect, both toward yourself and your client; about clear agreements that you make and live by.

Bobby's issue with Erica came from a sense that his personal integrity was being challenged. He had clear boundaries of appropriate behavior for himself and his clients, and Erica persistently tried to ignore them.

An analysis of integrity is really a disguised discussion about the self. For you to state what you stand for, a definable sense of your "self" needs to emerge. In all relationships, especially professional ones, letting the "other" know the rules, limits, and boundaries is mandatory. Then, as if your relationship was being played on a tennis court with its markings, you get to call the action as fair or foul. Going through the described process for making agreements will prove to be a useful tool for establishing minimum boundaries.

Figure 3.5: Sample Contract

Terms of Agreement

Date: _____

Parties to the Agreement:

_____   _____

What are you agreeing to do?

What am I expecting you to do?

When and where will these things take place?

What is the duration of this agreement?
From: ___/___/___   To: ___/___/___

What are my goals and objectives?

What are your goals and objectives?

What costs are involved?

When and how will these costs be dealt with?

What conditions or actions would make this agreement invalid?

Figure 3.6

Agreement Checklist

1. How do you feel about how you handled the meeting?
   OK _____   Not OK _____
   What would you do differently?

2. How do you feel about your client?
   OK _____   Not OK _____
   What bothers you?

3. Is there any important unfinished business?
   Yes _____   No _____
   If yes, what is it?

4. How clearly do you think your client understands what you will do and what you won't do?
   Very _____   Not very _____   Not at all _____
   What do you need to do about it?

5. How clearly do you understand your client's commitment to and awareness of the effort, risk, and potential payoffs?
   Very _____   Not very _____   Not at all _____
   What do you need to do about it?

6. How explicit were you in detailing the elements of your agreement (time, costs, penalties, limits)?
   Very _____   Not very _____   Not at all _____
   What do you need to do about it?

7. Where were you the clearest?

8. Where were you the least clear?

9. How, if at all, would you change the way you handled yourself or the terms of your agreement?

This may all seem simple to do. You may know yourself well enough to state your limits, rules, and boundaries clearly in virtually any situation. Or you may struggle in some situations to figure out where you stand. On occasion, you may even find yourself saying one thing and doing another.

It may be hard to take a stand, especially if your professional code of conduct is unclear or nonspecific. Yet, if an action doesn't feel right to you, trust yourself enough to check out your feelings and other reactions.

"Follow your bliss. There is something inside of you that knows when you're in the center, that knows when you're on the beam or off the beam. And if you get off the beam to earn money, you've lost your life. And if you stay in the center and don't get any money, you still have your bliss."

—Joseph Campbell,
The Power of Myth (1988)

Chapter 4

RESOLUTION:
UNDERSTANDING AND RESOLVING INTERPERSONAL CONFLICTS

*"Not everything that is faced can be changed,
but nothing can be changed until it is faced."*

—James Baldwin

The coach was like a desert wind blowing hot in the day, cold at night, and switching directions without warning. Rules were maybes, and threats were empty. Some thought he had favorites, but others believed his behavior was motivated by fears about job security. Eddie was late for practice. Coach Dubbins spotted him out of the corner of his eye. "Hey, Barnes, get over here," the coach growled. "Yeah coach, sorry, I had to talk to one of my profs after class."

Dubbins snorted. "Listen Barnes, this is twice this week. You know the rule—three tardies and you're on the bench for the next game . . . and if you're out of two games, you're gonna lose your ride!"

Eddie bowed penitently, "Okay coach. I'm really sorry. It won't happen again."

The athlete backed away and slid into practice at the foul line. Buzz wore a sly grin as he sidled up to Eddie and said "Coach chew you out again, Mr. Superstar?"

"Yeah, so what?" Eddie boasted. "He needs me more than I need him."

"Big talk, Eddie," Buzz responded. "You've got a full ride—you want to lose your scholarship, tough guy?"

"Look, Bozo," Eddie grinned, "without me, this team would be in last place."

Buzz stepped toward Eddie and poked him in the chest with his finger. Before Eddie could open his mouth, Jonesie hit him in the butt with the ball and broke the tension. Buzz retrieved the ball and dribbled off toward the basket. Eddie stood firm with hands on his hips, waiting for the next challenge. It didn't come.

Eddie was again late for Friday's practice. Coach Dubbins yelled across the court, "Barnes, go home! We don't need you. You're out of the game Saturday, but be there anyway." Dubbins turned his back as Eddie stormed toward the locker room. Buzz yelled after him, "Hey Eddie, don't forget to bring a cushion." The rest of the team laughed nervously. They knew what the game would be like without Eddie.

By half time in Saturday's game, the team was trailing 16 points. Coach Dubbins paced in the locker room. "What the hell's the matter with you guys? You're playing like you don't care who wins." He turned to Eddie who was sitting in the corner with a strained look on his face. "Look here, Barnes, are you part of this team or what? You're goin' in for the second half. We're countin' on you." A broad smile lit up Eddie's face. Buzz punched the locker so hard he cut open one of his knuckles. "What the hell's the matter with you, Buzzie Boy?" the coach mocked. "You wanna play on this team, then you play by the rules. And the rules are what I say they are. You got it?"

"Yeah, I got it, coach!" Buzz spat out the last word like a viper projecting venom. Dubbins let it pass as he turned back to Eddie. "And Eddie, if you're late again next week, that's gonna be it for you. You hear me?"

"Sure thing, coach." Eddie rose from the bench and muttered an aside to Buzz, "You can count on the coach to stick to his word. Right, Buzzie Boy?"

We see some strong conflicts in this story, and we also see that some of these conflicts get resolved—at least on the surface level. What remains at deeper levels will continue to affect the players as long as they remain in relationship to one another. So, we can easily predict that a new conflict (or an old one that was never fully resolved) is just around the corner.

Conflicts arise from differences, yet differences per se are often a natural and positive aspect of life. We will begin our discussion of resolution with an examination of differences and how they may develop into conflicts.

DIFFERENT STROKES FOR DIFFERENT FOLKS

Differences in approach or opinion are integral to life. They don't necessarily mean that something is wrong or that a relationship is in trouble. In life, it's wise to expect differences. They're natural and, depending on how you view them, can be positive rather than negative.

Differences can be important to personal growth and to the development of relationships. We need diversity to open us up to new possibilities, to novel perspectives, and to exciting opportunities. Isn't variety the spice of life?

THE ADDED ELEMENT OF CONFLICT

Conflict adds further dimension to differences by bringing in the element of struggle or competition. Differences come to be experienced as oppositional, rather than as neutral or benign.

Conflicts may range from minor disagreements over needs, rules, methods, or terms, to deeper clashes about purpose, values, or personality. They may stem from miscommunication, from perceptual discrepancies, or from real and intolerable differences. We may experience conflict as the feeling of "I'm right—you're wrong!" or as the conviction of "I want to win and, therefore, you have to lose."

In conflict situations something is at stake, and this something may be different from what you think it is. Although it may look as if pride or ego is involved, it could be your integrity. A boundary may have been crossed, an agreement broken. You may have experienced a violation of respect or fairness in the relationship.

MIXING POWER WITH CONFLICT

How we approach one another in a conflict may depend on perceptions of power: how powerful you perceive yourself and others to be, and how willing both parties are to share power.

Over the centuries, philosophers, statesmen, and poets have tried to define the essence of power. These quotations reflect varied perceptions about the concept of power and some of its apparent contradictions:

> "Knowledge itself is power." (Francis Bacon, 1561–1626)

> "He who has his thumb on the purse has the power." (Otto von Bismarck, 1815–1898)

> "Old as I am, for ladies' love unfit, the power of beauty I remember yet." (John Dryden, 1631–1700)

> "Power tends to corrupt and absolute power corrupts absolutely." (Lord Acton, 1834–1902)

> "Power is the ultimate aphrodisiac." (Henry Kissinger, 1923–)

> "The highest proof of virtue is to possess boundless power without abusing it." (Lord Macauley, 1800–1859)

> ". . . all power is a trust—that we are accountable for its exercise." (Benjamin Disraeli, 1804–1881)

> "No one is to be trusted with power." (Charles Percy Snow, 1905–)

> "Thou hast not half the power to do me harm as I have to be hurt." (William Shakespeare, 1564–1616)

> "The love of liberty is the love of others; the love of power is the love of ourselves." (William Hazlitt, 1778–1830)

> "Where love rules, there is no will to power." (Carl Jung, 1875–1961)

> "We thought, because we had power, we had wisdom." (Stephen Vincent Benet, 1898–1943)

> "Do not pray for tasks equal to your powers. Pray for powers equal to your tasks." (Phillips Brooks, 1835–1893)

> "Self-reverence, self-knowledge, self-control—

these three alone lead life to sovereign power.''
(Alfred Lord Tennyson, 1809–1892)

These quotes illustrate different interpretations of power. To some it is good while to others it is evil. Some believe power comes from inside the self or from your character, while others deal with power as an interpersonal phenomenon based on such attributes as beauty, money, or position.

Power Jargon

Present-day power jargon may confuse the discussion even more. People talk about power ties, power suits, power breakfasts, power lunches, power plays, and power cars. Is it true that if we wear particular clothes, drive certain cars, hold certain jobs, or speak with certain gestures, we will be perceived as powerful?

We fully agree that power is something others may perceive you have. Since the media urge us to think that possessing certain suits, ties, cars, or watches equals power, we may attribute power to people because of what they wear, what they drive, or how they talk. As a result we could be misled.

Perceptions of Power

Power isn't something you receive along with the keys to your new Lamborghini; it's what others may think you have because they might perceive you as richer or, in some other way, better than they—because you drive a Lamborghini.

If beauty is power, how much power does a beautiful woman have with a blind man? If money is power, how much power does money have with a Buddhist monk? If knowledge is power, how much power does an educated person have with someone who cannot understand her words?

Interpersonal power involves two people in an equation. John perceives something about Mary that causes him to let her influence his behavior. If John didn't perceive this or was indifferent to this something, he wouldn't let her influence him.

What about the extremes of interpersonal power? Power isn't just a matter of perception. You don't have to perceive a person's muscular strength for that person to be able to overpower you physically. An extremely wealthy person can also manipulate your life without your even knowing it. Some dimensions of another person's power are so extreme in relation to your own that you are rendered powerless to influence the situation. At most, you might only have personal power to influence your attitudes toward yourself.

Under more common conditions, we hope to find ourselves in situations were power is shared, not necessarily equally, but to a degree in which each person can influence the other's actions. How much each party can influence the other depends on the actual powers each person has, as well as the powers each perceives the other to have.

The Roots of Interpersonal Power

Interpersonal power has its roots in perceptions of giving and receiving. What kinds of things can people give you that you want enough to let them influence you? Here's a short but comprehensive list of reasons you let someone influence you to act in a certain way:

Reward: You perceive he will give you positive things or things you want—like money, a job, a promotion, an award—for your actions.

> Example: A person who offers you a high-paying job.

Punishment: You perceive she will do negative things to you—like firing you, taking something away, or reducing your status—unless you behave accordingly.

> Example: A coach who tells you to pass the ball.

Expertise: You perceive he has expert knowledge or skill that is better than what you have.

> Example: A physiotherapist who suggests a rehabilitation plan.

Information: You perceive she has information that you want or are lacking.

> Example: A staff attendant whom you ask for instructions on the cardio machines.

Acceptance: You perceive he has the ability to make you feel visible, loved, valued, or accepted.

> Example: An inspirational teacher who counsels you.

Legitimate Authority: You acknowledge that the person holds a certain office or position to which you are supposed to respond in specific ways.

> Example: The director of a health and fitness center where you work.

These descriptions of the roots of power

1. allow power to be a neutral concept, and

2. acknowledge that your perceptions of power could be inaccurate.

According to the first perspective, there is nothing inherently right or wrong with your taking a high-paying job, listening to the coach, or wanting to be liked by your teacher. From the second perspective, the staff attendant may not know how to work the cardio machines, but she gives you directions nonetheless. Your coach may be wrong. Your teacher may never make you feel valued.

Interpersonal power involves an exchange. Tom gives Joe something in return for something else. Elsa takes Sally's advice about a money problem because Sally is her accountant; Elsa pays Sally a fee. Once again, we're back to agreements, except now we have a clearer idea about the stuff of the agreement. You have expertise that you agree to provide in exchange for a reward of money. Is that all there is to it?

Conflict also relates to this discussion. How we behave in situations where there are disagreements or conflicts may derive from our perceptions of interpersonal power. If you don't get your way and you think you have power over the other person, you may be tempted to use it. The other person, perceiving you to be more powerful, may behave in ways contrary to her or his best interests.

How to Retain Your Personal Power in Conflicts

What has been missing from this discussion is what we reviewed in Integrity (Chapter 3). The give-and-take of relationships might be regarded within the context of boundaries. More centrally, we recommend that relationships in conflict be guided by four qualities: respect, understanding, caring, and fairness.

Interpersonal power becomes problematic when it is used to violate boundaries or to disregard the rights of self or others.

Life does not guarantee that others will always use power in respectful and fair ways. However, it remains within your personal power to conduct yourself with respect, understanding, caring, and fairness. You never need deprive yourself of these qualities in relationships with others or with yourself. Availing yourself of these qualities allows you to retain your personal power, your perspective on what is best for you to do, and your ability to make sound judgments about how to conduct yourself in conflict resolution.

Our goal is to show you how you can be successful, keep your job, and have as many clients as you need without giving your personal power (or yourself) away!

> **Key Point:** *No conflict is worth resolving at the cost of your self-esteem.*

POWER PLAYS

In the scenario at the beginning of this chapter, who had what kinds of power? Coach Dubbins may have had five kinds of power: reward, punishment, expertise, information, and legitimate authority. As school coach, he had authority to give or take away scholarships or even playing positions. Presumably, as an expert in the field he had the information that players needed to improve their performance. The power of the coach's acceptance would depend on whether a player cared about how the coach felt toward him.

Eddie Barnes's main form of power came from his expertise. He was talented, and coach and teammates needed him if they wanted to win. Eddie also might have had the power of information about the game. Finally, some of the players might have seen him as prestigious and would then let him influence them because they wanted Eddie to like them (acceptance).

Eddie didn't have much power with Buzz. Buzz didn't care whether Eddie liked him, and winning was less important to Buzz than maintaining his self-respect. On the other hand, Coach Dubbins influenced Buzz because Buzz wanted to play ball, and the coach could let him play or throw him off the team (reward and punishment).

It doesn't seem as if anyone in this situation retained his personal power or his self-esteem. Coach Dubbins went back on his word to win—he acted in an unfair manner and showed disrespect for his team. Eddie used his power to get his way rather than to live up to his agreement. Buzz tried to take a stand for his values, but in the end yielded to the coach's threat. Buzz thereby gave away his self-esteem.

ORIGINS OF CONFLICTS

Where did the basketball court conflicts originate? From one perspective, we can say the conflicts came from broken agreements. Eddie was on a basketball scholarship that carried with it certain responsibilities. He was also a member of a team that had at least an expectation of teamwork from the players and abiding by the rules. Eddie broke these agreements.

Coach Dubbins had an agreement with the players about overseeing their practice sessions and enforcing rules. He broke his agreement.

We might see Buzz as violating an agreement of team cooperation in that he hassled and mocked Eddie for being late. Even though Buzz's behavior may seem understandable, he too contributed to the team's conflicts.

MOVING TOWARD RESOLUTION

Resolving conflicts isn't about winning or being right. It's about negotiating an agreement in which both parties feel respected, understood, and fairly treated; clarifying terms and issues; and mutually determining the most equitable and satisfactory solution possible.

Does this sound possible? How could Eddie and the coach both be winners? How could Buzz feel good about what happened at half time on Saturday? Conflicts in this scenario were resolved through an abuse of power, not through fair-minded discussion and mutual decision making. Buzz harassed Eddie. Coach Dubbins made the decisions and then remade them. One could only assume what needs the different actors were expressing through their behaviors, and the assumptions of their needs tended to be negative: Eddie was a spoiled superstar, Buzz was a hothead, and Dubbins was unethical.

BUILDING ON SUPPORT, PURPOSE, AND INTEGRITY

Skills emphasized in previous chapters on support, purpose, and integrity contribute to the prevention of conflicts.

- Listening to people without getting defensive moderates the emotions in disagreements and allows you to hear the problems accurately and respond in a caring manner.

- Discovering what others want and being clear about your own purposes enable you to understand what's going on and are necessary to reaching fair agreements.

- Knowing your role, your personal boundaries, and those of your clients allows you to behave respectfully, that is, to respect your own values and needs and those of the people with whom you work.

- Referring to the terms of agreements helps clarify perceptions that may have veered off from what was originally decided and makes room for renegotiation where warranted.

Giving people support, knowing your goals and those of your clients, and respecting boundaries through clear and fair agreements will reduce the chances for disagreement, but all of this won't necessarily prevent disagreements. When conflicts arise, you will have even more need for these critical conflict-resolution skills.

Support in Conflict Resolution

Imagine that when Eddie showed up late, Buzz approached him and said, "Coach is really on your case. Is there anything I can do to help?" Eddie might have responded in the same arrogant, defensive manner, but he might have softened his attitude and let Buzz into his personal plight. Eddie's response could have sounded like this: "I don't know, Buzz, I've just got too much to do—and I'm cruisin' toward academic probation."

Being supportive during a disagreement means acting respectfully toward the other person and allowing her to say how she feels and what she needs.

- **Check your response:** Is it blaming, avoiding, minimizing, agreeing, or disagreeing? Do you fully understand the other person's issues in the conflict?

- **Mirror communications:** Let the other person know you understand. Tell the other person what you hear as her or his issues.

- **Ask for confirmation:** Ask whether your understanding is accurate before you respond.

- **Acknowledge agreements:** Acknowledge as often as possible where you agree—in truth or principle—with what the other person is saying.

Purpose in Conflict Resolution

When disagreements or conflicts occur, people may be acting at cross-purposes. Eddie may want to be the superstar to whom the rules do not apply, while Buzz may want to be part of a cooperative team. Perhaps one person's expectations of the agreement are not being met. These expectations may not have been dealt with up front, but they can still influence behavior. Coach Dubbins might never have made it clear that the rules applied only so long as his team was winning. He created conflict in the team by not living up to what team members perceived as his agreement with them. Eddie might have had a more realistic view of the agreement: He seemed to understand what Coach Dubbins's behavior implied.

When you become aware of a conflict or disagreement with another person, check your purpose and then the other person's.

- **Your purpose:** What purpose did you agree to? Is your purpose being met in this relationship? Have you made all aspects of your purpose clear to yourself and to the other person?

- **The other's purpose:** What purpose did this person agree to? How do you know whether the other person's purpose is being met in this relationship? What evidence might you have suggesting that some aspects of the other person's purpose remain hidden? Are you aware of aspects of the other person's purpose that were never agreed to, but are operating nonetheless? Are you playing a psychological game by occasionally satisfying the other's unstated purpose?

Let's return to Coach Dubbins and Eddie Barnes. Barnes has an agreement with the coach to play basketball. Eddie knows this, but his agreement has a condition he hasn't fully discussed with his coach. He wants a real education, so schoolwork is at least as important to him as playing basketball. Dubbins may only care that Eddie maintains the minimum scholastic standing of a C average. Eddie may have plans for graduate school and want a minimum of a B average.

Let's revise the dialogue between Coach Dubbins and Eddie:

Coach: "Hey Eddie, come here for a minute."
Eddie: "Yeah coach, I know I'm late. I'm sorry. I had to talk to one of my profs."

Coach: "Listen Eddie, I'm concerned. This is the second time you've been late this week, and both of us know you've been averaging two tardies a week ever since we started the season. . . . You know the agreement we have about your scholarship and playing on the team. What's happening, kid?"

Eddie: "I don't know what else to tell you, Coach . . . you're right. I'll just have to try harder."

Coach: "Eddie, it seems to me you want to try hard, but I get the feeling something's interfering with your getting to practice on time."

Eddie: "Well, you know coach, I've gotta keep up my grades. I'm having a hard time in some of my courses."

Coach: "Hard time? Like what's goin' on?"

Eddie: "Well, this is my last shot at pulling up my grades before I apply to grad school, and my first 2 years weren't so hot."

Coach: "I see, Eddie . . . I didn't know this. Now things are starting to make more sense."

Eddie and Coach Dubbins are really talking now, and they're getting at Eddie's unstated purpose. Knowing this purpose puts the coach in a much better position to help both Eddie and himself achieve their own goals. Compare this basis for action to one where Coach Dubbins assumes that Eddie just has a bad attitude or a chip on his shoulder.

Integrity in Conflict Resolution

Integrity is about boundaries and rules. One boundary crossed in the basketball scenario was a rule about coming to practice. Coach Dubbins was within his rights to impose a penalty on Eddie; however, his reversal of position at half time during the game represented a lack of integrity or ethics.

Eddie's integrity required him to talk to the coach before the situation got out of hand. He had agreed to certain behavior standards as part of his athletic scholarship; but he went over the line by showing up late. Yet, Eddie wasn't willing to sacrifice his future for the team's success. He had a higher purpose than winning the game. The athlete wasn't being fair and respectful to his future plans and to his agreement with the coach. In terms of integrity, Eddie was as much at fault as Coach Dubbins. Like the coach, the player violated his agreement to pursue something he deemed more important than his word.

How could things turn out all right for everybody in this situation? How would the coach and players get to maintain their integrity? The dialogue continues from where we left off.

Coach: "I see, Eddie . . . I didn't know this. Now things are starting to make more sense."

Eddie: "Yeah, I feel in a real bind. I know I'm not doing what I should for the team, but I feel caught."

Coach: "Eddie, tell me, what ideas do you have about solving this problem?"

Eddie: "Well, I don't know, coach. I've been studying real hard. It's just that some of the material is really beyond me. I guess if I'd gotten down the basics in the prereq courses, I'd have less trouble now."

Coach: "I see. So, you're missing some of the basics and that's slowing you down now."

Eddie: "Yeah, that's a big part of my problem. I'm just playing catch-up all the time, and it's getting in the way of my showing up."

Coach: "Eddie, I have an idea. You're not the first player who's had this kind of problem. Over the years, I've developed some real trust in an academic advisor in your department. Would you like me to give you his name?"

Eddie: "Sure, coach. If you think it'll help, I'd be glad to give it a try. I don't mean to be a problem. I know I'm not living up to my agreement by always being late for practice."

Coach: "I know that, Eddie. I'll give you his number after practice and I hope you set up a meeting as soon as possible."

Eddie: "Great, coach—and thanks! This means a lot to me."

Coach: "Hey, Eddie, we both have a lot at stake in this. You've got your scholarship, and I've got my reputation."

SKILL DEVELOPMENT FOR RESOLUTION: STEPS TOWARD RESOLVING CONFLICTS

Now that you have some appreciation for the dynamics of conflicts, let's consider the steps in an effective conflict resolution process. You may not need all the steps in the following process, or you may move through them at lightning speed, but each step can have critical importance. The whole process is well worth knowing.

Here are 15 steps toward resolving differences. Rather than trying to memorize them, work toward understanding what they are. We'll give you a checklist at the end that summarizes the steps and allows you evaluate your conflict resolution process in a particular situation.

Step 1. Clarify to yourself what the conflict is about. What do you think the conflict is? Determine what the issue is for you. Maybe the conflict doesn't really involve the other person, even though you feel as if it does. If the conflict does involve the other person, get clear about the issues.

Step 2. Decide whether it's worth confronting; if it is, decide how and when to confront it. Make sure the conflict is worth the energy you will invest in resolving it. Consider your goals and the relationship in making your decision. If the relationship is worth the effort you will invest in resolving the conflict or your goals are important, then figure out an appropriate time to address the matter. Remember: Effective conflict resolution takes time.

If the situation is one in which another person approaches you with a conflict, you can still decide whether you want to resolve it, or if this is a good time for you to deal with the conflict.

Step 3. Describe the other person's actions. Don't label, accuse, or give value-laden descriptions. Describe the other person's actions in a factual and accurate manner.

Accusatory: "You have been acting in an irresponsible manner."

Factual: "You were late for practice 3 days in a row this week."

Step 4. Define the conflict as a mutual problem. Avoid defining the conflict as a "right-wrong" or "win-lose" situation. Present the conflict as a mutual problem whose resolution will benefit both of you.

Win-Lose: "You're going to have to change your behavior."

Mutual: "This situation affects both of us so it would be good to figure it out together."

Step 5. Define the conflict as specifically as possible. The more general and nonspecific the definition of the conflict, the more difficult it will be to resolve. Work toward the narrowest and most specific definition of the problem.

General: "You have a real attitude problem."

Specific: "Not calling in when you're going to be late for work is the issue I'd like for us to discuss."

Step 6: Factually describe the effects of the conflict. What do you perceive to be the specific consequences of this conflict? These may include loss of time, money, energy, effectiveness, or morale. Beware of overwhelming the person with dramatic descriptions of consequences or, at the opposite extreme, of minimizing the impact of the problem.

Overdrawn: "Because of your behavior, the team has lost its motivation."

Underdrawn: "Your behavior is only hurting yourself."

Factual: "Your lateness for practice makes it difficult for some of the other players to get all the practice they need on plays where you're involved . . . and that may have a negative effect on team performance."

Step 7. Describe your emotional response to the other person's actions. Feelings are an important part of your reaction. Don't hide your emotions or expect the other person to know them.

Hidden: "You can imagine how this made me feel."

Open: "It angered me to have to stand around for a whole hour waiting for you to show up."

Step 8. Describe what you have done (or what you omitted doing) that helped to create or to continue the conflict. Conflicts are always two-sided. Maybe your inaction is your contribution to the conflict: You let it go on without saying anything; or, perhaps, you stated the rules ambiguously.

Denying your responsibility: "I've lived up to my end of the bargain. There is no way that I'm responsible for this problem."

Acknowledging your role: "I might have let you know sooner." Or, "Maybe I needed to write down my policy about lateness so there was no chance for uncertainty."

Step 9. Understand the other person's perspective. How does the other person see the conflict? Unless the two of you can come to a mutual definition of the conflict, you will be arguing about separate issues. Understanding the other's perspective requires mirroring skills. Not only do you need to hear what the other person has to say, but you also need to demonstrate that you heard the person accurately by reflecting her or his perspective.

Step 10. Reaching a mutual definition of the conflict. Perhaps you have defined a conflict that the other person didn't perceive to be a conflict. This is analogous to the other person's saying, "Well, that's your problem. I don't have a problem with that." If you have followed all the steps to this point, you will have communicated how the problem affects both of you and how its resolution requires the involvement of both of you. Before moving on to strategies for resolution, make sure you are both working on the same problem. Remember that until Coach

Dubbins and Eddie Barnes agreed to work on the same issue, they could make no progress in the situation.

Step 11. Generate potential solutions for mutual benefit. Generating potential solutions for mutual benefit requires an open mind and a belief that the solution is something you discover rather than something you know and are just waiting to impose. Potential solutions are also best when generated by both of you in a cooperative fashion, by asking for input from the other person. Also important is the use of brainstorming— the free-wheeling generation of suggestions without judging the feasibility of the ideas until the next step. The key features of the brainstorming process are to

- remain open-minded,
- involve the other person,
- generate as many options as possible, and
- delay evaluation of the options until you have finished brainstorming.

Step 12. Evaluate the potential solutions. Once all your ideas are in the open, you can evaluate the viability of the various proposals to resolve the conflict. In the example of Coach Dubbins and Eddie Barnes, the coach proposed a solution that Eddie would meet with an academic advisor. Eddie could have suggested other solutions, but this one seemed to hit the mark and was seized upon instantly. Conflict resolution sometimes works that way, but don't count on the first proposal you come up with (especially if it's yours) being the right one.

Step 13. Detail your mutual decision. Perhaps an ambiguous agreement brought you into the conflict. You want to be sure to cover all the bases in your agreement to a new solution. What do you need to specify? Does the agreement need to be written? What consequences will apply if the solution doesn't solve the problem, and when will those consequences come into play? All these details need to be thought about, discussed, and agreed to. You might wish to refer back to the section on Agreements in Chapter 3.

Step 14. Implement your solution. With the solution detailed and responsibilities assigned, you each can do your part to implement the new solution.

Step 15. Check on how it's going. Rather than assuming that all will be well now that you've dealt with the conflict and arrived at a mutually agreed-upon solution, it's best to target a follow-up meeting when you can check with each other on how the solution is working. We also recommend agreeing on a method to monitor the situation so it doesn't get out of hand in the future, or so you can catch it early on, if it spins out of control.

A Conflict Resolution Checklist

After you complete a conflict resolution meeting, the following checklist (Figure 4.1) might help you to determine whether you hit all the points or whether you left something out.

Did your answers to the checklist indicate that you skipped any steps in the conflict resolution process? Do you know why you omitted the steps? How can you improve your conflict resolution approach? Make notes about your ideas for future reference.

A REFLECTIVE SUMMARY

Conflict occurs whether we take an active role in it or not. Many times, it seems easier just to ignore conflict or to smooth it over in the hope it will go away.

Although conflict itself is not bad, it can become the reason for saying and doing things that make or break relationships. Often old hurts and hard feelings get put on the table along with the facts and issues. Being able to sort out emotional reactions from the facts of situations will help free you to enter the arena of conflict or disagreement.

Where does one get the perspective, the calmness, the tools to handle conflict? It is inside you. All you really need is your self—the one that results from accepting and respecting yourself. The more you accept and respect yourself, the easier it will be for you to listen to the other person, to be supportive even though you may not be in agreement, to work toward understanding how your purposes mesh and how they differ.

In conflict situations your being right doesn't automatically make the other person wrong. Just because others don't agree with you or cross your line doesn't mean they are wrong! It may be frustrating or upsetting, but on a practical level all that conflict resolution requires is that you deal with it. Even if you have repeatedly alerted another to a conflict situation in the past, effective conflict resolution may require you to assert yourself again and again. You may even have to change or end the relationship to maintain your personal integrity in the face of a persistent conflict.

Figure 4.1

A Checklist for Resolving Conflicts

After you complete a conflict resolution meeting, use this checklist to determine whether you hit all the points or whether you left something out.

1.	Did you clarify to yourself what the conflict was about?	❑ Yes	❑ No
2a.	Was it worth confronting?	❑ Yes	❑ No
2b.	Did you arrange to confront the person at a good time and under favorable conditions?	❑ Yes	❑ No
3.	Did you factually describe the other person's actions?	❑ Yes	❑ No
4.	Did you indicate that the problem was of mutual concern?	❑ Yes	❑ No
5.	Did you define the conflict as specifically as possible?	❑ Yes	❑ No
6.	Did you accurately represent the effects of the conflict?	❑ Yes	❑ No
7.	Did you accurately present your emotional response to the conflict?	❑ Yes	❑ No
8.	Did you describe your part in the conflict—what you have done or omitted doing?	❑ Yes	❑ No
9a.	Did you invite the other person to express her/his perceptions of the conflict?	❑ Yes	❑ No
9b.	Did you verbally reflect your understanding of what the other person said to you?	❑ Yes	❑ No
10.	Did you reach a mutual definition of the conflict?	❑ Yes	❑ No
11a.	Did you generate potential solutions for mutual benefit without prejudgment?	❑ Yes	❑ No
11b.	With the other person's involvement?	❑ Yes	❑ No
12.	Did you work together in evaluating the potential solutions?	❑ Yes	❑ No
13.	Did you work out all the details of your mutual decision?	❑ Yes	❑ No
14.	Did you fully implement your solution?	❑ Yes	❑ No
15.	Did you set up a time and a place to discuss how the solution is working?	❑ Yes	❑ No

Chapter 5

INSPIRATION: CONNECTING TO THE SPIRIT

"Don't be a magician, be magic."

—Leonard Cohen

Janet was on time, as usual. Her appointment with Lisa was always circled in red on her calendar, and barring the end of the world Janet would show up.

Over the years, Janet had tried many things to relieve her neck tension, her back pain, and her general feeling of incompletion. She didn't feel at home in her body and knew something needed to change.

On her worst days, Janet felt almost apologetic for not being happy. She thought she should just grow up and accept that this was all there was. On these days, she didn't have to look too far to find people to agree with her.

Janet had met Lisa, her massage therapist, at a wholistic health conference. Lisa's talk about the mind-body connection had sparked Janet's interest, and she made an appointment with Lisa the following week.

That was a year and a half ago, and through weekly sessions, Janet realized her first impression of Lisa had been accurate. Lisa's warmth, caring, and personal well-being were consistently present. Her hands moved directly from her heart. Janet imagined an angel had entered her life; she felt so fully received by Lisa.

Janet's body responded to Lisa's caring touch. As the months went by, Janet felt freer and more at home in her body. Even with these gains, her work was not finished. Janet continued to experience a lingering sense of incompletion. Lisa sensed that beneath Janet's physical tension was a person trying to fly, whose energy seemed stuck on the runway.

Lisa approached bodywork in a way that extended it beyond the weekly sessions. She listened to Janet's feelings; she came to understand the day-to-day pressures that served to disconnect Janet from her body. Lisa helped Janet find solutions that would support her throughout the week. The therapist recommended that Janet complement bodywork with classes in yoga and swimming. Janet acknowledged the need for expanded work and took the suggestions. Her body and mind thanked her.

The balance was gradually shifting. Janet felt closer than ever to what she had imagined years ago as only a vague possibility. And she knew that when that possibility entered her life, she would embrace it.

One day as Janet entered the studio for her weekly massage, she became aware of Lisa's excitement. Her smile spoke first.

After an enthusiastic hello, Lisa said, "Janet, I've been aware of something in my work with you lately, and I think I may have a perfect way to connect you to it."

Janet picked up on Lisa's contagious excitement and asked, "What is it? Tell me!"

"It would be my pleasure," Lisa said with a hint of pride. "I took a workshop last year from this incredible dancer. Actually, he's more than a dancer. He teaches dance that captures the spirit as I have never experienced it before. His classes are primitive, sensual, and uniquely expressive. And I just got a brochure announcing that he's coming here to teach for 6 months."

Janet took it all in and responded with an inner certainty that Lisa was on to something. "All right, Lisa, I've tried your other ideas, why not this one? It may be the piece I'm missing."

A couple of months later, Janet showed up for her regular appointment. She looked transformed, not so much in external ways, but in the sense of herself that reached out to meet you. This wasn't entirely new; It was just more perceptible than the week before and the week before that. And she had the most amazing news.

INSPIRATION OR JUST DOING YOUR JOB?

Is this a story about inspiration or about someone "just doing her job"? Our most optimistic answer to this is BOTH. Lisa probably did as much for all her clients, yet this quite ordinary behavior was nonetheless remarkable.

Lisa had deeply affected Janet's life. All she needed was for someone to support her as she got to the heart of the matter. Lisa really listened and, when needed, asked supportive questions. The care and respect Lisa demonstrated allowed Janet's submerged self-knowledge to emerge. Janet's trust for Lisa grew over time, and it enabled her to hear the wisdom in Lisa's words.

Where others had concurred with Janet's self-limiting beliefs, Lisa's approach allowed Janet to blossom at her own pace. No one performed heroic tasks. No rescue trucks were required. The magic fairy dust stayed in the bottle. Lisa offered simple qualities of acceptance and support. Janet already had what she needed to actualize her dream—it was inside, waiting to be born. Lisa helped Janet move from discouragement to possibility and then to "amazing news."

Flying Lessons

How often kids say, "I wish I could fly," only to be met with reasons why they can't. What if more people responded with "Tell me more about it. I remember feeling that way." Or, "Fly? What would that be like for you?"

What if each of us brought to our work a commitment to encourage clients' beliefs in themselves?

Where did Lisa learn to be inspirational? Did she discover the ingredients with the help of an inspirational teacher or guide or an Obe Wan Kenobe telling her to believe in herself? Perhaps her parents turned mundane chores into play and adventure, encouraged her dreams, and helped her see the possibilities of reaching them.

It's unlikely family ties would get all the kudos for Lisa's inspirational abilities. Some credit certainly goes to her personal life experiences— whether early or late—that guided and rewarded her efforts to be herself. It's also likely that Lisa's studies incorporated the value of self-care. It would seem a necessary lesson if she was to take on the responsibility of caring for others.

If we were offered a behind-the-scenes look at Lisa's life, we would likely see a person who takes good care of herself. We would find her asking for support when she felt she needed it and choosing goals that reinforced her purposes in life. Even though she works in a hands-on field, she would manifest a clear sense of where she ends and the other person begins. Her efforts to make boundaries clear and respectful would shine through in her behavior toward others. Even amid the emotions of conflict, we would see her approaching situations with a win-win attitude.

And what would be the result of this process of nurturing and respecting herself? We believe it would be the capacity to be inspirational to herself and to others.

The Thunderbolt That Stays

You may think of inspiration as a thunderbolt kind of experience, or as a cartoonish lightbulb going on in your head. That's one sense of the term, but we have chosen to use it differently. We like the "sustained thunderbolt" interpretation of inspiration.

Lisa didn't stand on a soapbox and give Janet an inspirational speech one day or put a secret decoder ring in the bottom of her cereal box. It was far more subtle—and sustained. It was her way of being with Janet over time that made the difference, not one critical sentence or one flashing insight. From time to time Lisa really connected with Janet and offered her some perception or a suggested path of action. Yet it was the persistence of Lisa's support, the consistency of her caring, the nonjudgmental way she continued to believe in Janet's native wisdom that ultimately worked magic.

Do Fairy Tales Come True?

The word inspiration has its roots in Latin, meaning "to breathe [life] into." We see it clearly in fairy tales where someone breathes life into another: Geppetto and Pinocchio, the Prince and Sleeping Beauty, Beauty and the Beast, the Wizard of Oz and the Tin Man.

Are fairy tales so different from your personal experiences of inspiration? At different points you may have felt discouraged, doubted yourself, or felt directionless. Some part of you was lifeless or asleep. Then, you met someone who inspired you, who breathed life into you, who enabled you to believe in yourself and your process of becoming real. You felt a real relationship with this person—no matter how long it lasted. You became visible, alive, valued, and bursting with potential. This relationship didn't require the fireworks of July. It represented a moment of truth, carefully nurtured, protected, and sustained in its infancy and early development.

Lisa was present to Janet's inherent possibilities. She honored her process of growth, no matter how difficult it may have seemed in the moment. She provided Janet with the necessary space to resolve her doubts and appreciate her purpose. Lisa helped Janet plug into the magic that was inherently hers.

BECOMING INSPIRATIONAL

Remember the scene in *The Wizard of Oz* where Dorothy and her companions discover that the wizard is a fake? Ironically, in this discovery they receive the greatest gift of all. The wizard gives them symbols for what they inherently possess—a clock for the Tin Man's heart, a medal for the Lion's courage, and a diploma for the Scarecrow's native wisdom.

They had what they needed all along. What prevented them from knowing it was the belief that they were lacking or undeserving and that to get what they needed, someone else had to give it to them; they were unable to see and acknowledge what was within them.

Are we asking you to be the Wizard of Oz? Yes! And what magic tricks or symbols do we think you have to give? You can start with respect, understanding, caring, and fairness, first for yourself and then for the other. You have no need for special fairy dust or extraordinary feats. Just being real with yourself and extending this realness to others will enable you to become inspirational.

Carpe Diem! (Seize the Day!)

Maybe you don't have a wizard or a Lisa in your life and think you have to wait for one before you can become inspired. Unlike the fairytale characters you are not under a spell, and you don't have to wait. We are here to help you along the way. In the previous chapters you have already taken steps toward the "self" knowledge you need on the journey to inspiration. Keep following the yellow brick road.

A good way to continue is by taking the best possible care of yourself. If you're waiting to do this, do you know why? Are you waiting to believe you deserve it? Are you waiting until you've finished taking care of everyone else? Or, are you waiting until someone tells you you're worth taking care of? Don't wait. Begin today—with you. Inspire yourself with the value you place on your self.

The journey doesn't stop at the self. Being inspirational to others will develop out of the time you invest in discovering your purpose, defining your boundaries, and learning your limits. It will come from challenging self-limiting beliefs and affirming yourself and will grow through addressing your conflicts and resolving them as best you can at this point.

Becoming inspirational is a process. Maybe you're well on your way or perhaps started in some aspects of your life. For most of us, the process is an ongoing life journey. We value and respect your work in progress and hope this book breathes life into it.

SKILL DEVELOPMENT FOR INSPIRATION: SELF-ACTUALIZING BELIEFS

How we think about ourselves, situations, and others greatly affects our feelings and our ability to be inspirational. Often, our fears and other feelings overwhelm us, and in the rush for comfort, we automatically envision ourselves, others, and life as wrong (or negative). Eventually we may become one with these beliefs, even if they don't reflect our true selves. In this section we discuss facing, challenging, and transforming self-limiting beliefs.

Beliefs can be either self-limiting (negative) or self-actualizing (positive). You ask a friend to take a step aerobics class, and he declines your invitation with an apology: "I'm not very coordinated." His belief limits him from participating, and it further reinforces his attitude that he can't. You could argue with him that aerobics doesn't require much coordination or that he is coordinated enough, and you might continue to encounter his resistance. You might be able to bully him into taking the class, but he would probably prove his point by tripping over his feet.

Is this a case of stubbornness or is there something else going on? We believe that if you spent more time with this friend examining the beliefs under his beliefs, you would discover a fundamental belief of the variety, "I'm just not good enough." Beneath this belief, you would likely find fear.

Perhaps you hear an argument growing inside you that sounds like this: "Are you trying to tell me that if he believes he can't do step aerobics, that he has a core belief that he's not good enough in general?"

Yes, that is what we're saying. What prevents this person from taking the class and tripping over his feet or having a good time despite being out of step with everyone else? Is it embarrassment? Self-confidence? Self-acceptance? Did his fears and self-limiting beliefs demand that he say no?

This person could have said, "I don't want to take step aerobics right now" without the slightest implication of not being good enough. Remember, he says, "I'm not very coordinated." He asserts something negative about himself.

He could have said lots of other things:

- "I enjoy challenges—I've never done it but am willing to try."
- "I feel a bit self-conscious, but I'm willing to learn."
- "I've done more difficult things in my life. Why not?"
- "Sounds like fun."
- "I can do that!"

Believing in oneself is usually a matter of degree, rather than an all-or-none phenomenon. The same friend who says he's uncoordinated may also say, "But I'm a great runner." In this statement, he asserts a positive belief that he thinks may balance his negative belief. This approach treats our self as a kind of balance statement between our assets and our liabilities, our pros and our cons, our positives and our negatives.

Rather than take this balance sheet perspective, we prefer to accentuate the positive and, moreover, to reframe what your mind wants you to believe are negative or limiting sides of your nature.

Attitude, Acceptance, and Affirmation: The Triple-As of Self-Actualization

The triple-As of reframing negative or self-limiting beliefs as positive ones that promote self-actualization are

- attitude,
- acceptance, and
- affirmation.

Step 1. Identify negative attitudes. Begin with the negative attitudes or beliefs you have about yourself, such as "I'm clumsy and uncoordinated," "I have bad luck," or more generally, "I'm not good enough." These attitudes are self-limiting beliefs that create obstacles to being your best. These attitudes may arise from judgments about your feelings. You might take a feeling like the anxiety you experience as you're about to deliver a speech and turn it into a self-limiting belief, such as, "I'm an incompetent public speaker [because I feel anxious when I speak]."

Step 2. Accept yourself. Self-acceptance is a prerequisite for changing attitudes and beliefs. You acknowledge your feelings and resist turning them into negative, self-limiting beliefs.

You are a person in process, not a fixed identity. You evolve throughout life toward actualizing all of you. Right now, you may experience anxious feelings. Rather than making these feelings into unchanging beliefs that lock you in place, such as, "I'm incompetent," acknowledge your feelings as momentary and choose to embrace a more positive view of yourself. This view can be expressed in an affirmation.

Step 3. Affirm your self. All the resources you need to realize your potential are within you. An affirmation activates qualities you already possess. Even when you doubt these qualities, persistent repetition of self-affirming statements realigns your course toward positive growth. Affirmations don't counter feelings—they counter negative beliefs. Affirmations are vehicles of change that move the very best of you forward. To see how this happens, let's move deeper into the semantics of affirmation.

Personal, Present, and Positive: The Triple Ps of Affirmation

Principles for forming self-affirming beliefs can be summarized in the triple Ps:

> **p**ersonal,
>
> **p**ositive, and
>
> **p**resent.

Personal: Affirmations begin with "I." Rather than saying, "People are good and trustworthy," say, "I am good and trustworthy."

Positive: Self-affirming statements are positive. They move you toward optimal possibilities and define paths to "self-actualization." Your affirmation may be a new thought that switches old emotions from reverse to forward drive, like taking fear and using it as fuel for positive change. Statements of affirmation disallow negative ideas, or even negations of negative beliefs, such as, "I'm not clumsy" or "I'm not incapable." Instead, these statements assert, "I am . . ." You can fill in the blank with words like strong, healthy, caring, confident, capable, loving, successful or with phrases such as, in control of my life, able to achieve my life's ambitions, or respectful, fair, caring, and understanding.

Present: The third *P* refers to time, and the time is now. Affirming statements are about the present. They aren't in the form, "I will become a good person" or "I used to be caring." They assert the very best of you in the now. "I am competent." "I am good enough, right now!" "I have all I need to be successful in this moment."

What if, when walking onto a stage to give a speech, you are aware of feeling anxious? Remember that anxiety is a feeling, not a fact about who you are. You can feel anxious, acknowledge this feeling, and at the same time affirm that you are competent and can handle the situation.

The Triple-As Take Patience

Hang in there! And breathe! When strong feelings come up, it means they're on their way out. Your mind may resist your statements of self-affirming beliefs—and that's okay. Continue your affirmations. Beliefs are the product of conditioning. In time and with practice, you'll condition new beliefs—ones that are positive, life affirming, and self-actualizing.

And What About Dorothy?

The Wizard of Oz was able to inspire everyone except Dorothy. She wasn't missing a heart, courage, or a mind; she was missing Kansas. Because the wizard had no words or ticking clocks that could help Dorothy get there, he offered to take her there himself. Yet as the story goes, that didn't work out. The wizard couldn't really do it for her; Dorothy had to do it for herself. She felt devastated and saw no way out.

At this critical juncture, along came Glinda, the Good Witch. She reminded Dorothy that all she needed to get back home to Kansas was to believe she could. And we know how that turned out. Dorothy repeated her affirmation (not her wish) three times, and it became a reality. The words "There's no place like home" and a click of the ruby-red shoes transported her to a place she had never really left. This brings us to the final point of the story.

Dorothy had been operating on some strong negative beliefs about herself, her life, and others. Unless you believe she really went to Oz, all that happened to her was that she changed her attitudes, and this process allowed her to be aware, alive, and grateful. Home became a wonderful place—inside and outside.

A REFLECTIVE SUMMARY

We don't think it's necessary to believe in magic to appreciate the effect one person can have on another.

When we encourage clients to find that place inside that feels real (like "home") and they do, it enables them to make choices in positive self-affirming ways. Our clients will begin to commit to life and health for reasons that are positive, rather than to support negative beliefs such as "I am ugly" or "I can't . . ." or "I have to . . ."

To inspire, to breathe. Each breath we take is inspirational. It is a choice, an affirmation, an assertion that "I am. . ."

"I breathe, therefore I am!"

Chapter 6

TIMING: OPPORTUNITY KNOCKS

"To every thing there is a season, and a time to every purpose under heaven."

—Ecclesiastes 3:1–8

Jeff took a deep breath as if to ready himself for action, but instead of meeting force with force, he merely shrugged his shoulders. His slow exhalation signaled what might be interpreted as defeat, yet it wasn't. Hank's eyes flashed in defiance, and then he walked away, muttering, "It's a stupid rule—I'm going to talk to the manager . . . then we'll see what happens." He brushed Jeff's shoulder as he passed.

"What's that all about?" Eve whispered.

"Ah, it was nothing," Jeff replied as he struggled inwardly to ground the electrical charge coursing through his body. Hank was young and a bit hot-headed. Jeff didn't need to justify Hank's behavior—he just couldn't take him on right now. The club was crowded, and a big row was the last thing anyone needed. Members had been in foul humor all day. Maybe it was the full moon or the bad economy or the post-Christmas blues. Whatever it was, Jeff didn't have the energy to enter another debate about the club's policy allowing only 30 minutes on the cardio machines. Hank had exceeded the limit, and the lineup behind him was growing impatient. Asking Hank to get off the machine wasn't easy, but it was part of Jeff's job.

Amid his reflections, Jeff noticed the aerobics instructor storming out of the classroom. She was yelling, "I'm not teaching in there again. It's too darn hot. And the sound system's screwed up."

Her class stood immobilized, not knowing whether she would come back or whether someone else would fill in. Jeff quickly caught up with her.

"Hey Sandy, wait up a second. What's goin' on?"

"Jeff, I just can't teach here anymore. The room is a mess. It's too hot and the sound system won't work!"

"I hear ya," Jeff sympathized. "Can I do something to make it better for the next hour, and then we can take a closer look at the situation after class?"

"What can you do?" Sandy challenged.

"Oh brother," Jeff thought to himself. "She's finally had it. Be cool. This is no time to chime in with your own version of 'I've had a bad day, too!'"

"Sandy, I'm real sorry about the problems. . . . Your students are waiting for you right now. Let me crank up the air-conditioning and open a few windows for you. What's wrong with the sound system?"

"I can't get the speakers to work. That system is so old. I always have trouble with it!" Sandy said in an accusatory tone.

"I think I know how to fix that, Sandy," Jeff replied in a way that sidestepped her blame. "Could you give it a try, Sandy, if I work on the speakers and the air for you?"

"Oh, all right!" Sandy conceded, "but this is the last time! I need that temperature adjusted before I start my class—not at the last minute!"

Jeff nodded empathically. "I agree, Sandy, and thanks for going back. We'll get together right after class to figure out how to avoid these problems in the future."

As Sandy strode back into class, Jeff thought, "Well, that was a good decision. No sense in reminding her it's her responsibility to check the music and air before class. Even so, they should have replaced that sound system long ago, and the floors could be kept cleaner. I think Sandy and I need to talk to the manager about this situation, but for now, I better get the air-conditioning working."

IT'S ABOUT TIME!

We could say, "It's all about time." The importance of time and timing is evident in sports, running a race, catching a ball, executing a dive. Time and timing also play an important part in human relationships, but in this realm they may seem more mysterious and less subject to slow-motion study.

No matter how great an idea you have, if it's the wrong time, it won't be heard. You may know exactly what to say, but if the listener isn't receptive, your message may be ignored. If you move too quickly in a relationship, you may find yourself at its end before there's a chance for a middle. If you move too slowly, a relationship may never develop beyond its initial level. And if you're not there at the right time, life goes on without you.

We have divided our discussion of timing in relationships into three interrelated themes:

- **Timing and intervention:** The first theme is represented in the interactions between Jeff, Hank, and Sandy. This sense of timing has to do with the broad question, "What intervention is most appropriate at this time?"

- **Timing and reliability:** The second theme is about reliability and the need for predictability, for example, being where you agreed to be at the designated hour.

- **Timing and relationship passages:** This aspect of timing has to do with the changes relationships may go through over time. Your ability to move at a rate appropriate to the relationship's development will be a key ingredient in your success.

Timing and Intervention

"What intervention is most appropriate at this time?" We said this was a broad question because it encompasses a number of smaller questions:

- What's your role?
- What are your resources?
- What's the situation?

By now this material is familiar ground. Let's examine Jeff's two principal interactions from the perspective of his role, resources, and the nature of the situation. We'll be answering the question, "Is this the right time?" but we'll add to it a further query, "For what?"

What's Your Role?

Jeff was an assistant manager at a fitness center. His duties included overseeing members' activities, assisting staff trainers, enforcing club policies, and troubleshooting in general. It was his job to remind Hank of the 30-minute rule and to request that he turn the machine over to another member. It was also his job to help with unexpected problems that instructors might encounter. Sandy's problem represented a minor emergency—it required immediate action. A long-term solution to her problem would require the manager's intervention, but at the moment first aid was needed. Based on his role, Jeff's action was appropriate and timely.

What Are Your Resources?

Resources not only have to do with facilities, equipment, and the availability of other people, but they also pertain to you in the moment. In the opening scenario, Jeff had been dealing with a lot of upset people that day, and, based on previous encounters with Hank, may have had difficulty distancing himself emotionally from Hank's aggression. On really bad days, you may be governed by the last-straw principle, losing control at a point when you are least able to deal effectively with the consequences. When your personal resources are at an ebb, you have to pick your battles carefully and handle what you can.

Jeff showed wisdom in avoiding a further confrontation with Hank. It may have looked as if he wimped out to Hank, but as the saying goes, "Discretion is the better part of valor." What would Jeff have accomplished by letting Hank engage him in battle? Jeff may have lost his cool—and Hank as a member.

Where did Jeff find the energy to deal with Sandy? We can only speculate about the answer. Perhaps he felt he had to deal with the problem because no one else could—and the class was waiting. Jeff was, in effect, a scarce resource. Perhaps his own feelings were less entangled in the situation with Sandy than in the one with Hank, so that he felt more resourceful in that moment.

Jeff could have done a number of things with Sandy, including ignoring her, blaming her, or referring her to the manager. Fortunately, he knew how to get the air-conditioning going and fix the speakers. Without these resources, Jeff would have had to fall back on resources outside himself.

You may be responsible for something, but if your personal resources are quickly dissipating, you may need to be creative in how you invest your remaining energy. Sometimes this means being absolutely clear about where you are in the moment. Imagine Jeff was completely at the end of his rope and Hank was known to get "snarky" when confronted. Jeff might then ask another staff trainer to do the police work while he took over a less taxing duty.

You may not be able to control someone else's behavior, but you do have the option of taking yourself in hand. You may not be able to control when another person wants to be mad at you, but your response belongs to you. Ask yourself:

- How prepared am I to take on the issues this person is presenting?
- What are my resources at this moment?
- Would there be a better time to respond?

What's the Situation?

Jeff acknowledged that the situation with Sandy needed to be dealt with immediately or else it would get worse. The situation required his physical assistance; it was not the time to review an instructor's job responsibilities. In the situation with Hank, he recognized Hank's volatility and focused on the task at hand, namely, getting Hank off the machine.

In appreciating situational dynamics, it helps to be clear about your goal. The question, "What intervention is most appropriate at this time?" implies you have a particular goal in mind.

Key Point: *Knowing your goal is essential to identifying what the time is right for.*

Jeff's interaction with Hank was goal oriented: He wanted Hank off the machine so another member could use it. A secondary goal might have been to re-educate Hank concerning the consequences of abusing this time-limiting rule. If Jeff had engaged Hank with this secondary goal, he might not have been successful, because the situation was stacked against it. The club was crowded. Tempers were short. And Hank was known to be belligerent. There would be a better time to accomplish this secondary goal.

Jeff's interaction with Sandy also had a primary goal, to get class under way. Again, we can see Jeff's secondary goals of bringing about a long-term solution to the sound-system problem and reviewing Sandy's job responsibilities. The situation wasn't right for this secondary goal. A discussion of job responsibilities and repairing equipment takes time. It can't be effectively accomplished while a class is eagerly awaiting the instructor.

Timing and Reliability

In a wonderful passage from *The Little Prince* by Antoine de Saint-Exupery, the fox admonishes the Little Prince for arriving unexpectedly. He tells him, "If you come at just any time, I shall never know at what hour my heart is to be ready to greet you. . . . One must observe the proper rites." The fox describes the importance of rites: "[Rites are] actions too often neglected. . . . They are what make one day different from other days, one hour from other hours."

Reliability and Personal Freedom

Knowing when certain things take place allows for predictability in life. Regional competitions occur at a particular time of year. Baseball has its season. The moon has its cycle. Academic courses have their term. Our calendars have hours scheduled for appointments. We depend on these rites or schedules to organize our lives and to create a sense of personal freedom.

Being professional means being predictable in certain ways, notably about time. Schedules bring security. You don't always have to be thinking about what's happening next. You can relax and get into a rhythm. You also create this sense of predictability and rhythm for those with whom you work. This may sound like rigidity, but it's not at all what we're suggesting. To be spontaneous and creative, we need a context. Unless creativity has established boundaries, what we create may appear chaotic.

Are we really helping others when we are always open to being rescheduled? People may want us to be flexible, but is that always a good idea? Does it benefit another if we extend the time we have allocated for a meeting or if we are always willing to adjust our appointments?

Your Reliability Means Their Commitment

The locker in a local health center has a large sign hanging over the door: "Showing up is 88% of life." Commitment is partially demonstrated by showing up at practice or working out on a regular basis. We would like to make more evident how health/fitness professionals create the context for others' commitment.

Put yourself in the shoes of an athlete who is working hard to succeed. The athlete's performance is roughly equated with his or her self-esteem. How well she shoots baskets this morning or how well he runs in practice will affect how the athlete feels the rest of the day.

As this athlete, you look for certain emotional anchors in your competitive world. You're a little anxious as you walk into the gym, but then you see your coach. He's there with a welcoming smile and a friendly "How's it goin'?" You feel more anchored. You enter the locker room and are greeted by the athletic therapist, who's there as usual but today wants to know, "How's the knee? Feeling any better?" Your anxiety starts to disappear. You're in flow—into the routine. Without labeling it or knowing it, your coach and the athletic therapist have created a context for your commitment. Their timing—their presence in a predictable way—enables you to ground yourself in this reality, and to channel your energy toward your goals.

Similarly, imagine you are a fitness club member who has belonged to the facility for over a year. It's still not easy getting there some days, but you do it. Today, your energy is low. As you enter the club, the receptionist greets you with a big "hello." Your energy isn't up to hers, but you respond in kind. One of the trainers pats you on the back as she walks by. "Hey, good to see you!" she says with a smile. You imagine she says that to all the members, but so what—it feels good. After you change, you drag your body into the weight room where a staff member greets you. The two of you talk about the weather for a few minutes and gradually the conversation drifts to what you are doing today. You start with an "I don't know" and then elaborate with a little help from the staff member. As you shower at the end of your workout, you marvel at the transformation. How did it happen? How did you get from feeling like a slug to doing an hour plus of pumping iron? Maybe it dawns on you that those warm welcomes, those predictable presences in your workout world facilitated your commitment. Their being in their places—"at the appointed hour," as the fox would say—let you know you were in your place, the right place for what you needed.

You might think, "I know people who are 'always there' who would make me feel a lot better if they weren't!" You're right. It isn't just being there—it's also the quality of your presence. Timing is only one of the six elements of SPIRIT.

Timing and Relationship Passages

Throughout this book, we have referred to timing in relationships by implying that relationship passages need to be respected.

In their simplest form, we can consider the passages of a relationship as the beginning, middle, and end. We know that what happens on a first date is likely to be quite different from interactions between the couple a few months later. Actions considered forward or presumptuous at one point may come to be expected later on.

How do we become sensitive to relationship passages? How do we know when it's okay to discuss certain matters, or when we need to keep our own counsel? There are no simple answers. Our progress toward learning these subtleties of communication will be enabled by constructive feedback from friends and colleagues.

SKILL DEVELOPMENT FOR TIMING: "PLEASE, NOT NOW!"

We hope you have gained perspective about well-timed actions, the "when to . . .," through your reading of earlier chapters. There are also some general guidelines for "when NOT to" discuss, confront, or interact. We offer you this "when NOT to" advice as our further reflections on the boundaries of behavior.

We suggest you think twice about interacting when . . .

. . . the place or location is inappropriate to the nature of the conversation. If an issue properly belongs between you and one other person, keep it there. Don't expose it in public. This includes interactions like giving someone constructive feedback, discussing personal issues, or even providing exceptional praise.

. . . the costs (emotional, financial, etc.) are likely to outweigh the benefits. Imagine that you have considered the problematic situation, and you perceive that dealing effectively with this issue would take far more energy, time, money, or other resources than you presently have available. Further, you recognize that the outcome of any action would be insignificant or small in proportion to what you would have to invest. The interaction between Jeff and Hank demonstrates this point clearly. It would have taken Jeff far more energy than he had to help Hank feel okay about the time-limit rule—and the benefits would have been too small to justify the interaction.

. . . your goals for the interaction cannot realistically be achieved in the time you have available. We believe a common human error is to raise significant issues with another person as you are walking out the door. Another mistake is bringing up in a conversation more issues than you have time to discuss adequately. Check your watch first. If you don't have enough time to settle an issue, make a date for a future meeting when there will be time.

. . . you are unclear about your agenda. You have some vague feelings of discomfort or nagging thoughts that you can't quite identify, so you engage a client in conversation to help you focus more clearly on what's at issue. In this interaction, you are likely to convey your discomfort as well as a sense that you're beating around the bush because that is, in fact, what you are doing. However, in this case, even you don't know what you're trying to get at.

. . . *you are unable to distance yourself emotionally from the agenda.* We're not suggesting you must have solid control of all your emotions before engaging in a dialog; however, sometimes our emotions are so much ahead of our thoughts that they have the potential to totally direct our behavior. In this situation, a little time out or a period of reflection might help you feel more centered.

. . . *you are experiencing difficulty in establishing or maintaining your boundaries.* Perhaps you are confused about your role in a situation, or you sense that the other person is relating to you in a manner that conveys very mixed signals about what he or she thinks your role is. At the very least, slow the action down. Gather more information before responding. Figure out what your place is in the scenario. And, take time out if needed.

. . . *your need to win or be right feels stronger than your need to solve the problem.* This case resembles the previous one, except that one aspect of your emotional state is clear: You feel a strong desire to be right or to win no matter what. If this happens to you, take time to think things over, to sleep on it, or even to break for a water fountain trip.

. . . *the other person is not acting in good faith.* When another person is behaving in good faith in relationship to you, you are likely to feel respected, understood, cared for, and treated in a fair and equitable manner. Without making judgment about why someone you are dealing with does not appear to be acting in good faith, we suggest you recognize the absence of these feelings as ill omens for the moment. Perhaps these behaviors will change in time. If not, then there may be no right time for this relationship.

SKILL DEVELOPMENT FOR TIMING: BEGINNINGS, MIDDLES, AND ENDINGS

It's easy to find articles describing the various phases in different types of relationships. Magazine and newspaper items typically describe love relationships as beginning with "infatuation," moving through phases like the "honeymoon," and then plateauing in something like "mature love."

We can simplify this progression by thinking of relationships as having beginnings, middles, and endings.

In the Beginning. . . .

Walk respectfully toward the other, allowing time and ritual to deepen your working relationship. At the outset, you will gather information that will enable you to unlock the doors to the other person's inspirational energy, commitment, and personal integrity. You will learn how to be most effective in enabling the other person to achieve his or her goals. This is the time when you will find the places where you connect with the other, as well as where you are separate. You will watch for signs inviting you to come closer or telling you to remain at a certain distance.

It's okay to take your time, to go slowly in the beginning. If you are reliable in your behavior, if you respect your needs, and if you allow the other person room to develop in her or his own time, your relationship will grow according to its needs.

In the Middle . . .

As the relationship develops, you will probably sense an easier rhythm. Through your efforts to be supportive, you have helped him discover purpose. You have respected his boundaries and effectively resolved conflicts as they have arisen. You have enabled him to discover his inspirational energy. As a result, he has developed a greater sense of ''self''—of independence. He moves straightforwardly toward his goals. His commitments to health, wellness, and physical activity take hold—and your own role in the relationship begins to shift.

If you start to feel less essential to his goals, it is to be expected at this stage. Encourage his independence. Your role in his future endeavors is due for reevaluation. You will need to review how you work together perhaps, and to establish new terms of agreement.

Key Point: *What is needed at one stage of a relationship may be unnecessary at another.*

Let's track a couple of relationships to see how behaviors that might not fit at the beginning more readily find room in the middle of the relationship.

The Second-Place Champ

Karen met the coach with averted eyes and a weak handshake. "Well coach, I'm really glad you took me onto the team—I sort of follow the old Avis motto, 'I may be second best, but I try harder.'"

Coach Jennings smiled supportively and welcomed Karen to the first team workout. She felt tempted to respond to Karen's comment about being second best but decided to see how this attitude manifested itself.

Weeks went by and the volleyball team drew close to its opening game. Jennings noticed that Karen's "Avis syndrome" showed up in different ways. Sometimes Karen had a clear shot at the ball, but would let someone else take it. Sometimes she would argue more strongly for another person's value to the starting lineup than for her own. During locker-room conversations Karen could often be heard apologizing for one thing or another. Yet this seemed to be only part of Karen, for she also made some of the most spectacular plays the coach had ever seen. The coach decided it was time for a little chat.

"Karen, I've been watching you closely over the past few weeks and wanted to talk to you about your role on the team in the upcoming season," Coach Jennings opened.

"What do you mean, coach? I've been playing real hard. . . . I know I could improve, but I'm really trying," Karen responded defensively.

"Whoa, hold on Karen. It's nothing like that. I think you're terrific. You're one of the best players I've seen in a long time," the coach replied.

"Coach Jennings, are you pulling my leg?" Karen appeared genuinely surprised.

The coach looked squarely in her eyes and said, "I mean it, Karen. I am truly impressed with your skill—and your teamwork. In fact, the only thing that confuses me is that I keep getting glimpses of you where you're putting yourself down or acting like you really are second string."

Karen's mouth dropped open. "I do that? I guess I always knew I was a good team player, but I never thought I was star material. My older sister had that honor, and maybe I thought there was only one star to a family."

"Karen, I hate to disillusion you, but you are the star on this team," Coach Jennings asserted. "Do you think you can live with that?" she added.

"Coach, are you saying I'm not Avis any more?" Karen said half smiling.

"That's right, Karen . . . and I'm not asking you to go around with a swelled head . . . but I do think it'd be a good time for you to start living up to your talents."

"Okay coach," Karen smiled broadly. "I think I can get used to that."

We can see an example of timing that respects relationship passages in the way the coach tracked information relevant to an important theme, Karen's self-perception. In the beginning, Coach Jennings had little to go on. Maybe Karen was second-string material. Even if the coach knew about her potential, confronting Karen on the first day of practice might have driven her self-effacing attitude underground. She might have felt that she would have to watch what she said, while still feeling the same way she had. The coach earned her right to comment on Karen's behavior. She never minimized Karen's feelings, she encouraged her to play her best, and she rewarded her efforts. The time was right to move the relationship forward.

The Perfect Client

Most of Ellen's clients regarded themselves as exceptional cases. They seemed to have the perfect alibis for not working out hard, for canceling at the last minute, and for needing a vacation from training every 6 weeks. But Wally was perfect. He never canceled, always showed up on time, and worked hard to achieve his goals. What could be better?

Wally was easy, a real pleasure to work with. At 42 he had been an out-of-shape couch potato and a former fitness dropout. Eleven months of training with Ellen had transformed him. His body fat was down to 16%, he had muscles, and he really seemed to enjoy training. Some days, Ellen would outline the workout, and Wally would say something like, "Oh yeah, Workout #3, I know it by heart." Without further prompting, he would start moving through the program.

Ellen looked forward to her hour with Wally. He was upbeat and regularly praised her work. She didn't have to figure out how to drag him through a workout or how to motivate him with new exercises because he got bored. He was the predictable calm in her day.

Yet, Ellen sensed a growing uneasiness in herself the last few times she trained Wally. She remembered that one of his original goals was to be able to work out on his own. Even though he was a terrific client, she needed to help him work on this goal as much as she helped him with the others.

Ellen scheduled periodic reviews with her clients as part of her practice. Wally's review was coming up, and she thought this would be an ideal time to confront the issue of his working out alone.

"Wally, I wanted to take a few minutes today to review our work together," Ellen began. "You've been training with me for nearly a year now, and I'm aware of how much progress you've made."

Wally winked his eye. "Yeah, it's great! I feel like a new man."

"Wally," Ellen continued, "you seem to know all our workouts by heart, and most of the time, you run through them practically by yourself. You've achieved your body fat objectives and, as I've told you during the free-weight sessions, your form is terrific."

Wally beamed. "Ellen, you make it sound so good, I'm beginning to wonder if there's a 'but' in this?"

"Not at all, Wally," Ellen said evenly. "I wanted to take this time to review and to set new goals with you. I know that when we first met, you said that eventually you'd like to be able to work out all on your own. Where do you see yourself in relation to that goal today?"

Wally pulled back slightly. "Huh . . . well. . . ." His eyes drifted up toward the ceiling and he began stroking his beard. "Well," he continued, "I really like working out with you," but Ellen heard something like doubt in his voice.

Ellen nodded, "Wally, I like training you, too, but I wonder how this fits with your original goal of being on your own in your training?" As soon as the words were out of her mouth, part of her wanted to retract them immediately. What was she doing? Wally was the perfect client, and here she was suggesting that maybe he didn't need her. Was she crazy?

"Listen Ellen," Wally finally said with more certainty in his voice. "Maybe you're right. I've made so much progress with you that I think I've become almost superstitious. I'm afraid if I don't have you around, I won't work out anymore."

Ellen exhaled slowly. "Wally, it's really up to you. I just feel that if that's still your goal, we could talk about a training schedule that'd help you reach your objective. For example, you might want to work out with me every other time and see how that goes. If it works, fine. If not, we can always change it back. What do you think?"

Wally paused for a long while. Then, a grin spread across his face. "Ellen, you know, your idea is beginning to grow on me. . . . It sounds like a good way to test my self-motivation, and I'll still have a chance to check things out with you. Who knows? I might get to a place where I can really rely on myself to be regular about exercise!" The thought gave him obvious pleasure.

Ellen smiled back. "Yeah, I can see that happening, Wally. You have a lot of self-motivation from what I've learned about you."

"Thanks, Ellen. That means a lot to me." As they finished the review, Wally grinned slyly, and said, "So what is it today, Workout #6?"

"Right on, Wally—you know it!" Ellen replied.

This scenario illustrates a transition in a relationship. Wally was such a great client that his objective of becoming independent in his training could almost slip by. Fortunately, Ellen's professional style included a periodic review of goals with her clients. When we like working with someone, we may risk encouraging his or her dependency on us. Ellen bit the bullet and raised the issue. Initially, Wally was surprised. Perhaps he had become too comfortable in relying on Ellen. Just as Ellen worked on his other goals, she also reminded him of his goal of moving toward independence.

Endings in Problematic Relationships

Health/fitness professionals may need to initiate endings of problematic relationships. It's difficult to identify all the elements of conversations leading up to these endings, but we wanted to give you some ideas about how to close relationships where

- you can no longer be supportive,
- you are at cross-purposes,
- your integrity is jeopardized,
- conflicts are unresolvable,
- the relationship saps your inspirational energy, or
- the time just isn't right.

You have worked throughout this book to understand the elements of **SPIRIT**. Consistent with these elements, endings might reflect these ideas:

- *Support:* You may want to show support for the other person by acknowledging and mirroring communications in this process of ending.

- *Purpose:* The ending needs to reflect either the ending of your purpose in working together or a divergence of your purposes such that you are unable or unwilling to accommodate the other person's purpose.

- *Integrity:* The ending process may provide opportunities to clarify boundary issues and to reaffirm the other's sense of wholeness.

- *Resolution of conflicts:* Sometimes conflicts are too large to resolve. In other cases, you may have tried to resolve the problem with unsatisfactory results. Even so, aspects of this process will be useful in managing emotionally charged endings.

- *Inspiration:* Ending the relationship can nonetheless be inspirational both in the way you do it and in the self-esteem you encourage in the other through this process.

- *Timing:* Recognizing that endings are important human events means that you work toward creating the time and the right circumstances to raise the issue. You want to be sure it doesn't come across in the manner of "Oh, by the way . . ."

In the examples that follow, we have created responses that include the difficult words that need to be said when ending a relationship. We have assumed that you have brought the issue up and have also assumed that in prior discussions you have been supportive and tried to be understanding.

Hard Ending #1: The Chronically Late Client

"I have come to a decision about working with you, and I'd appreciate it if you would hear me out. We've discussed the issue of your lateness a number of times. I've been clear with you that I can't work under these conditions. The situation hasn't improved. I appreciate the fact that you've tried to stick to our agreement, yet I need to discontinue our working together."

Hard Ending #2: The Persistent Suitor

"I need to tell you something, and I would appreciate if it you would listen to me carefully. I've told you before that I was not interested in going out with you on a date. You've continued to ask me out or to try, in some way, to turn our training sessions into dates. [For example] I've told you how uncomfortable this makes me feel. I've also told you I have a strict policy about not dating my clients. I understand this has been difficult for you to accept, yet I have to honor my decision. I need to end my working with you, for professional reasons.''

Hard Ending #3: The Insulting Client

''What I have to say is important, so I would appreciate it if you would listen to me carefully. This will be our last session together. I will no longer work as your physiotherapist. I mentioned to you before how much it bothered me when you made jokes about my ethnic background. You've stopped making comments to me, yet you have continued to make racially derogatory statements about others while we are working together. I can no longer condone this behavior by continuing to work with you. It isn't relevant to me why you do this—what matters is my personal and professional boundaries. Based on these, I have decided not to continue working with you.''

Hard Ending #4: The Athlete Who Didn't Make the Grade

''I think you may know where this conversation is leading. We've talked many times about your performance level, and I've indicated that it's not at the place that I need my athletes to perform. I realize you have tried, that you have really put yourself into the practice sessions, and I know how very much you want to be on the team. I think we have run through all the remedial possibilities, and your performance still hasn't come up to team level. I am officially taking you off the team. I regret this situation and would imagine you have to be feeling pretty upset also. If there is any way I can be supportive to you at this time, my office is open to you.''

Hard Ending #5: The Disruptive Student

[The fitness class has just ended.] ''Do you have a few minutes? I need to talk to you. We've talked before about your behavior in class that I find very disruptive. Since your behavior hasn't changed, I need to ask you to please not attend my class any more. I assume you are clear about my reasons—if not, I'm willing to tell them to you again.''

Hard Ending #6: The Client Who Needs a Couch

''I've reserved the last 10 minutes of our session today to tell you about a decision I've reached. I've been training you for about 6 months and am no longer comfortable with our time together being used as a counseling session. I've stated my feelings about this before, and your needs remain the same. I respect your need for someone to talk to, yet this is not my job. If at a future date you decide to pursue your fitness goals, I hope you will consider rehiring me.''

In the End

Once upon a time, movies were over when the screen flashed "The End" and cartoons ended with "That's All, Folks!" Now, we may find ourselves staring at a screen with rolling credits, still wondering how the story is going to end or perhaps even what happened. No one rode off into the sunset, no one "won," heroine and hero didn't live happily ever after, and truth and justice didn't triumph.

Some endings in the health/fitness world seem entirely natural and allow you to prepare for them. Sports have their season. The last game ends. Players move on to graduation or to retirement. The awards banquets, the farewell parties, and quiet talks about past and future allow room for feelings to be expressed, for thanks to be given, and for goodbyes to be acknowledged for what they are.

Athletes may devote years, if not decades, in preparation for one shining moment. Whether it's the Olympics or another showcase of excellence, the moment comes—and then it's over. The athletes go home in victory or in defeat, some to renew their effort, others to choose a new life path. The aftermath of ending requires much respect and consideration.

Perhaps in a less dramatic fashion, the best class ever arrives at its last session, and all the participants have trouble saying goodbye. Or the athlete, now fully recovered from injury, thrusts his hands in the air and cries, "No more physio . . . but thanks. . . . I couldn't have done it without you." The door closes and a silence envelops the space, but only for a moment—just before the door reopens showing a new face, a stranger, to be met, to be understood, to be helped, and then to be released.

Some endings take you by surprise. Your favorite client fails to show and won't return your calls. A promising player gives up. An old-time club member doesn't renew. An athlete makes a wrong move and ends her career. Because these endings are less foreseeable, are they of less significance? We don't think so, although they may be harder to address.

Much of your work as a health/fitness professional will be geared toward creating positive transitions and good endings. You work hard with your team to have a good season. You help your clients generate all the inspirational energy they need to become independent and self-reliant in their exercise programs. You devote yourself fearlessly to the recovery process of injured athletes. You throw yourself tirelessly into others' pursuits of that shining moment. Even when things don't develop as you had hoped, your work is still about making transitions and endings as good as possible.

The really great news is that our work as health/fitness professionals doesn't end when the relationship does IF we have encouraged another SPIRIT. Positive energy is contagious: SPIRIT doesn't end just because the game is over, the workout is finished, the injury is healed, or a career is in transition. It just gets passed on.

A REFLECTIVE SUMMARY

Timing is knowing when to intervene; when to listen and when to ask the next question; when to suggest change and when to reestablish boundaries; when to confront and when to say goodbye; when to be there for others and when to be there for yourself.

Developing this sense of timing is not as hard as it sounds. We've given you some guidelines to use along the way, and if no clues seem apparent, rely on the **SPIRIT**.

Chapter 7

SPIRIT IN ACTION:

A DAY IN THE LIFE

Eve lay in bed in the predawn light. Sleep passed into wakefulness as she found her mind drifting back to a conversation from a month ago. She still remembered Dennis's words. He had been her second appointment of the day, and she was feeling as if it were midnight. Dennis asked, "Eve, are you feeling all right? You seem tired." In the moment, Eve tried to deny it, pulling on her reserves to turn the session around. The ruse didn't work—at least not for her. She could no longer deny she was running on empty.

Eve had chosen her profession because it represented everything she loved and wanted to do. What had gone wrong?

Vitamin supplements seemed like the first good idea. Maybe she was just a little run down. She watched her diet a little more closely and noticed how she had gotten into the habit of wolfing fast food while on the run between clients. Sure, it was healthy fast food, but eating while racing across town in rush-hour traffic would give anyone indigestion.

The more closely she looked at herself, the more she realized that vitamins and dietary changes weren't going to be enough. In her efforts to be the very best for all those in her life, she had neglected giving herself the caring and respect she needed. Change was definitely in order.

She asked herself all the vital questions she posed to new clients and came up with a list of needs she had been neglecting. She knew she had to create a new game plan for her days that would make room for these needs, a "total fitness plan" for the complete fitness instructor!

Eve reached for the alarm on its second beep. Aware of her day's schedule and the promise she had made herself, she gently kissed her husband, Adam, good morning and began her day.

She made herself a banana smoothie and headed for the sun porch that also served as her summer office. Her mind switched into forward gear as she reviewed her appointment book. Now that she had a framework for the day, she put down her yoga mat and began 30 minutes of deep stretches. She finished with a 10-minute meditation, during which she repeated to herself the affirmations she had recently created to support her self-care. This was how to begin her day!

She interrupted her brisk walk to the fitness center to stop and buy a card for Adam. Tomorrow was their second wedding anniversary.

Eve entered the center and found herself instantly attracting hellos, hugs, and questions. Her smile was contagious, and she usually had a warm welcome for all.

Changing in the locker room brought her into contact with many of her new and old clients. Even though it was going to be difficult for her to decrease some involvements on the personal side of her role as personal trainer, she was motivated. Today's first test of her resolve appeared in a client who insisted on trying to engage her in conversation.

Fran said, "But Eve, I just need to ask you one little question. I need to know what your opinion is about vitamin supplements." Eve sighed as she responded, "Fran, I'm sure that's important to you, yet I am unable to talk right now. I'll see you Tuesday at noon, as scheduled." Eve could hear Fran complaining to Ruth as she left the locker room.

In spite of Fran's reaction, Eve felt good about standing up for her needs. She had a nine o'clock appointment, and she wasn't going to be late. Making her boundaries about time stick wasn't easy, yet it was critical if she was going to maintain her personal value about respect and caring.

Some of her clients thought their time with her had no end. They wanted her to be "on call," and she had often found herself in exactly that position. But that was last month's story.

Stan was waiting for her. He watched as she approached and prepared his sensual "hello." They had been working together for about 6 months, three mornings a week. Typically, on Monday morning Stan wanted to talk about his escapades over the weekend. It almost seemed this was a higher priority than his training. Today, she thought she would be ready for him.

"Hi, Stan. Ready to train?" she asked with conviction in her voice.

A bit taken aback by the force of her words, Stan tried to reply in kind. "Sure, of course."

"Great!" Eve responded. "Let's get going with some stretches." Eve moved deliberately toward the empty aerobics studio.

Stan thought this was his cue. "Oh, before we start, let me tell you this juicy story about what happened last night," Stan said.

Eve knew she had to speak up now. Taking a deep breath, she said, "Stan, I understand you'd like to tell me about your evening's adventures, yet I must again request that this time be limited to training and discussions about training."

"Well," Stan said defensively, "I thought that's what we were doing!"

"I understand you feel that way, Stan, and even if we could train while you talked, it is still unacceptable to me to listen to your sexual adventures," Eve said with only the slightest hint of nervousness in her voice.

Stan seemed to step backwards, although in fact he did not move. The surprise on his face gave way to a look of confusion, and then to upset for having ignored all of Eve's milder requests for him to stop this behavior. "Eve," he said, "I'm sincerely sorry. You're right . . . you had asked me nicely a number of times. I won't do it again."

"That's great, Stan," Eve replied with a smile. "Let's get started." The hour went smoothly and ended with a warm handshake.

Before her 10:30 a.m. appointment, Eve went into the employees' lounge and had a cup of tea and the fruit-and-bran muffin she brought from home.

Next on her agenda was the noontime aqua-fitness class she hardly considered work. The 12:00 p.m. session was so much fun. She had turned a routine water aerobics class into a combination chorus line tryout and water tag game.

Eve changed into her running gear right after class, despite the many attempts to engage her in conversation. During her run, she couldn't decide what made her feel better—running or having created the time to do it.

She showered after her run and dressed for her afternoon appointments. As she walked through the employee lounge, she saw Jeff, looking as if he was in a funk. Eve decided to ask, "Hey, Jeff, what's on your mind? You look deep in thought."

Jeff looked up, half relieved to be pulled out of his personal quandary. "Oh hi, Eve. I didn't even see you come in. I guess I was a bit lost in thought." The furrows in his brow remained, even though he tried to act more with it.

"Jeff, a penny for your thoughts?" Eve inquired lightly.

"That sounds like a deal. I'd be glad to get them off my mind," Jeff said with more visible relaxation of his face. "I've been trying to figure out what to do with Sandy."

Eve reflected, "Figure out what to do with Sandy—you mean the aerobics instructor?"

"Yeah, Sandy who teaches the evening class. Is it okay for me to ask you to keep this conversation just between the two of us?"

"Sure, I can agree to that." Eve responded with sincerity.

"Thanks," Jeff said. "Okay, here goes. The other night there was this little crisis involving Sandy. She kinda lost it and stormed out of her class. I helped put her and the class back together again, and that was great."

"So what's your concern?" Eve interjected.

"Well, I've been stewing about how to deal with her about the way she talked to me. I mean, I felt really disrespected." Jeff paused with another sigh. "I didn't like her taking her anger out on me, and I feel as if I need to tell her that."

"I hear you loud and clear," Eve said sympathetically.

"I'm upset with her for dumping on me," Jeff continued, "even though she had a point about that old stereo system. . . . I'm nervous about talking to her because I don't want it to escalate into a yelling match."

"Now, I understand what's got you so preoccupied. That does sound like a problem," Eve consoled. "But if you don't mind hearing my opinion," she continued, "I've got a few thoughts on the matter."

"No, I'd be glad to have your ideas, Eve. Go ahead, shoot!"

"Well, I don't know if it's shooting," Eve said, hoping that Jeff would understand this second meaning. "First of all, I think you have a right to your feelings, and you needn't let those feelings get in the way of your talking with Sandy. I also support the idea of your talking to her about this. I think it'll help you feel stronger self-respect and allow Sandy a chance to say, 'I'm sorry!' "

Jeff looked as if a large weight had been taken off his shoulders. He said, "Eve, thanks for understanding . . . and for your ideas. I feel more confident about talking to her now."

"I hope it goes smoothly for you," Eve said as she turned to leave.

"You're a real lifesaver," Jeff said genuinely.

Eve left the lounge feeling good about having helped a colleague. In the midst of the warm afterglow, she heard a tiny voice in the back of her mind asking, "Hey, Eve, did you really have the energy for that? Or was that just you taking care of someone else before yourself?" She continued walking around the fitness complex and soon found herself on the basketball court dribbling a ball and shooting hoops. It relaxed her and cleared her mind. The best she could figure was that she couldn't answer the question. It felt good to help and, yes, it took some energy. She wasn't Superwoman, so she agreed with herself to keep monitoring her energy and her decisions to get involved. It was the promise she had made herself, and it fit her affirmation of "I take care of myself first and have energy left for others."

Her last appointment of the day was a new client, who had been referred to her by one of her old clients. This would be a good opportunity to initiate some of the decisions she had reached about what was to go into her agreements with clients. Her new motto was "Be up front about time and money." Larry brought Gina to her office, and Eve welcomed her with a smile and an introduction. "Hi, I'm Eve and I'm glad you decided to work with me. Please make yourself comfortable."

Gina sat down and immediately began talking. "I'm glad you have time to work with me because Hank spoke so highly of you. I worked with another trainer for awhile, but she tended to be late all the time and it really bothered me."

Eve nodded but chose not to respond at this time. Instead, she began her interview process. "Gina, maybe we can start with your telling me what you'd like to get out of our working together."

Gina thought for a minute and then replied, "Well, you know, the usual things. I want to look good, and I'd really like to feel stronger. Become a bit tougher. You know."

"Well Gina, you've trained before, so you've had experience with the fitness world. Are there any activities that you've come to enjoy and might like to continue?" Eve inquired.

Gina sat up a bit straighter and said, "Actually, there is. I really love weight lifting. I'm not crazy about the machines, but I get a real kick out of working with free weights."

"Great." Eve said, smiling to herself about how Gina's desire to feel stronger tied in perfectly with one of the psychological benefits of weight training. "Is there anything else you might like to do?" Eve asked.

"Well, I'd like to be a better swimmer. Would you be willing to help me with swimming? I love being in the water." Gina paused, noticing how closely Eve seemed to be listening to her.

"Gina, I think we're going to be a good match. My real passion is the water. As a matter of fact, I teach an aqua-fitness class at lunchtime that sorta resembles a group of kids at recess. I'd love to help you with your swimming, and I'll help you design a weight routine that should give you what you want," Eve said.

"Super, I brought my stuff. Could we get started today?" Gina asked.

"Absolutely. As soon as we finish drawing up our agreement, we can change into bathing suits and begin in the pool." Eve reached into her desk and took out a contract she had created especially for personal training. "I'd like to go over this form with you and review what we shall be agreeing to."

After covering details of scheduling and program design, Eve reminded herself that she was worth it, and she forged ahead into the nitty-gritty of time and money. "Gina, I want to address the issue about lateness that you mentioned earlier, and present my rules about time and money. First of all, I want you to know you can depend on my side of the agreement, especially in regard to time. Our appointments are for 1 hour, and that hour begins at the scheduled time. Barring some unavoidable crisis, I'll be here at the time we agree to, ready to work in a manner I consider both professional and worthwhile.

"I also want to tell you about my policy with regard to any changes in our appointments. If you must cancel and you do so more than 24 hours in advance, there are no consequences. But if you miss an appointment or cancel with less than 24 hours' notice, I require full payment."

Eve stopped herself from saying more, resisting the temptation to explain or justify herself. She waited for Gina to respond.

After a long pause and a couple of "mmmm's," Gina spoke up. "Well, at least you're being very clear, and I think I can live with your policies." She paused again, then continued. "Actually, I think I respect you more for valuing yourself like this. That's the kind of tough I want to get."

As Eve finished with Gina, she knew she had done the right thing. Although there might have been misunderstanding and resentment between them around issues of time and money, she now felt as if she was both taking better care of herself and being fair with Gina. All in all, it felt like a day well spent. What she needed now was to unwind and reconnect with her husband.

She headed for the manager's office and was happy to find Adam at his desk. "Hi, honey. Do you have a free moment?" Eve asked.

"Hi, sweetheart. Boy, it's good to see you. What's up?" Adam responded.

"Well, I just finished my last appointment, and I'd love to make plans for us to have a very private, cozy dinner. I have a lot to tell you about my day, and I really haven't heard much about the workshop you took last weekend," Eve said, while relishing how much she had in common with Adam.

"You must have read my mind," Adam said. "How about 30 minutes to get ready, and then we'll go to your favorite place."

Eve was delighted. "Sounds perfect. And after dinner I want to read you the dedication in that wonderful book you bought me. I think the authors really understand the meaning of caring." Eve smiled at Adam, knowing he would agree.

A REFLECTIVE SUMMARY

Eve represents you. She works in the health/fitness professions, and she gives enormous energy to clients—often too much.

Her awareness of the need to take care of herself came during one of those overspent times, a time when she needed an outside boost to jump-start her battery.

Her awareness required action. She reviewed the situation, set out a plan, and let her internal voice be her battery check. She knew the issues: time, boundaries, and personal life. Eve had a lot going for her, and she needed some of it for herself. She needed to replenish the "source" and to put out clear messages that she was in charge of her life. The more she reinforced that "self," the more solid and clear she became in her relationships.

Eve came to live the **SPIRIT** of this book. She began with herself, and then, like a waterfall spilling over, she passed her extra energy on. Eve felt inspired by her choices and commitments, and so did her clients and her colleagues.

Is this possible? The choice is yours. Review where you are. Get a reading on your attitudes, your approaches, your agreements. Start with yourself. Listen to the messages on your "machine" (a.k.a your mind). Change the tapes that make you wrong, last, or not "good enough." Stop trying to run on low. Take the time, the courage, and the heart to live life as fully and joyfully as possible. Draw lines with such clarity that anyone crossing them would expect a trespassing ticket. Get nervous, get real, and get all that's available for the risking.

Perhaps your plan needs to include people who will cheer you on in the pursuit of your needs. Surround yourself with people who make you feel like clicking your heels and repeating the words that will take you home. . . to yourself.

Whatever paths this book takes you on, we wish you a safe, joyful, and wondrous journey.

INDEX

ABOUT THE AUTHORS

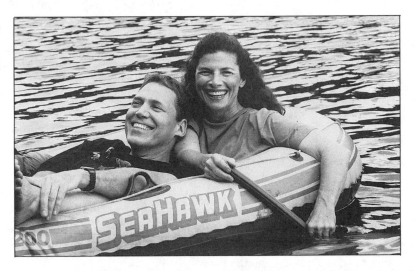

James Gavin has been a university professor and practicing psychologist since 1968, specializing in health promotion and counseling psychology. He earned his doctorate in psychology from New York University in 1969 and was awarded the Diplomate in Counseling Psychology by the American Board of Professional Psychology in 1984. Since 1980, Jim has been a professor of applied social science at Concordia University in Montreal. In keeping with his beliefs about health and exercise, Jim has been a competitive swimmer, triathlete, modern dancer, aerobics instructor, and yoga teacher.

Nettie Jane Gavin has a private practice in body-mind integration therapy, specializing in holistic transformations. She earned her master's degree in public administration from the University of Pittsburgh in 1975 with a concentration in group dynamics. A student of healing arts since 1974, Nettie has studied transpersonal psychology, yoga, t'ai chi, aikido, meditation, polarity therapy, and Kripalu bodywork.

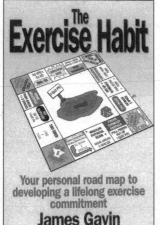